....

Obesity and Binge Eating Disorder

....

Bibliotheca Psychiatrica

No. 171

Series Editors

Anita Riecher-Rössler   *Basel*
Meir Steiner   *Hamilton*

KARGER

....

Obesity and Binge Eating Disorder

Volume Editors

Simone Munsch   Basel
Christoph Beglinger   Basel

33 figures and 13 tables, 2005

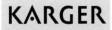

KARGER

Basel · Freiburg · Paris · London · New York ·
Bangalore · Bangkok · Singapore · Tokyo · Sydney

Bibliotheca Psychiatrica

Formerly published as 'Abhandlung aus der Neurologie, Psychiatrie, Psychologie und ihren Grenzgebieten' (Founded 1917)
Edited by K. Bonhoeffer, Berlin (1917–1939), J. Klaesi, Bern (1948–1952), J. Klaesi and E. Grünthal, Bern (1955–1967), E. Grünthal, Bern (1968), E. Grünthal and Th. Spoerri, Bern (1969–1971), Th. Spoerri, Bern (1973), P. Berner and E. Gabriel, Wien (1975–1986), B. Saletu, Wien (1986–2003)

••••••••••••••••••••••

Dr. Simone Munsch
Universität Basel
Institut für Psychologie
Missionsstrasse 60/62
CH–4055 Basel (Schweiz)

Prof. Dr. Christoph Beglinger
Abteilung für Gastroenterologie
Universität Basel
Petersgraben 4
CH–4031 Basel (Schweiz)

Library of Congress Cataloging-in-Publication Data

Obesity and binge eating disorder / volume editors, Simone Munsch, Christoph Beglinger.
　　p. ; cm. – (Bibliotheca psychiatrica ; no. 171)
　Includes bibliographical references and index.
　ISBN 3-8055-7832-6 (hardcover : alk. paper)
　1. Compulsive eating. 2. Obesity.
　[DNLM: 1. Obesity–therapy. 2. Bulimia–complications. 3. Bulimia–psychology. 4. Bulimia–therapy. 5. Obesity–complications. 6. Obesity–psychology.] I. Munsch, Simone. II. Beglinger, C. (Christoph), 1950- III. Series.
　RC552.C65O24 2005
　616.85′26–dc22

　　　　　　　　　　　　2005001671

Bibliographic Indices. This publication is listed in bibliographic services, including Current Contents® and Index Medicus.

Drug Dosage. The authors and the publisher have exerted every effort to ensure that drug selection and dosage set forth in this text are in accord with current recommendations and practice at the time of publication. However, in view of ongoing research, changes in government regulations, and the constant flow of information relating to drug therapy and drug reactions, the reader is urged to check the package insert for each drug for any change in indications and dosage and for added warnings and precautions. This is particularly important when the recommended agent is a new and/or infrequently employed drug.

© Copyright 2005 by S. Karger AG, P.O. Box, CH–4009 Basel (Switzerland)
www.karger.com
Printed in Switzerland on acid-free paper by Reinhardt Druck, Basel
ISBN 3–8055–7832–6

Contents

Contents

....

Preface

After lurking in the background for many years, overweight and obesity have relatively suddenly, on the scale of human disease, become a major problem affecting many countries across the world. The reason for this is the remarkably rapid increase in overweight and obesity in both children and adults. The problem in childhood is the most alarming statistic because the disease burdens associated with overweight and obesity are now projected to increase steadily in future years. Hence, obesity is a chronic disease associated with much morbidity and mortality. It is also a complex disorder with multiple biologic and environmental inputs controlling energy balance. Clearly the odds are against us at present because the human condition is tipped toward energy conservation and the present food and activity environments are pushing the weight curves to the right, although whether the whole population or only a (large) proportion of the population is involved in this trend is debatable at present. The environment is in control at present. In some countries today, the situation is reversed with too many people chasing too few calories. The result is that there are few obese individuals, or to put it more accurately there are fewer individuals who used to be thin, and many thin individuals who used to be overweight or obese. Both an abundance of food and starvation are excellent examples of the environment interacting with, and overwhelming, genetic predispositions.

Does a complex disorder always demand a complex understanding of the inputs from genes to environment and their various interactions to affect a cure? As Rees pointed out in a paper titled 'Complex disease and the new clinical sciences' published in *Science* in 2002, pernicious anemia is a complex disorder 'Yet once mechanistic insight was obtained, treatment was simple; injection of the missing vitamin B_{12}.' The Achilles' heel of the disease had been discovered. Clearly we have not yet discovered the Achilles' heel of overweight and obesity. Perhaps we never will, although at least for severe obesity, bariatric surgery, as described in this book, is close to such a simple approach, by cutting down on available calories in a way that appears acceptable to the majority of those affected.

Certainly, as this volume indicates, we have made many advances in our understanding of overweight and obesity in every area from the control of feeding and energy balance, to epidemiology, and to improvements in the various treatments available for these disorders. Yet despite these advances, the 'epidemic' as some now call it, is gathering speed. One of the most persistent problems is helping individuals to control their weight for health reasons is the lack of maintenance of weight losses in most studies that follow their participants for long enough. This brings us back to the problem that both biology and the environment are acting against weight loss in most developed countries. Because we can only control the biological pressures to a small extent, the focus should probably be on modifying the environment. If this is to be done well it would have to involve many levels of society from government, to the food industry, to the family. In other words, a well-organized public health campaign, somewhat modeled after the very successful efforts made to reduce the frequency of smoking.

The history of binge eating disorder (BED) is both separate and intertwined with that of obesity. Basically, once anorexia nervosa (AN) and bulimia nervosa (BN) were clearly defined, including their subclinical variants presently denoted as eating disorder not otherwise specified (EDNOS), it became recognized that there may be another eating disorder, often but not exclusively associated with overweight or obesity, characterized by binge eating without compensatory behaviors. The pros and cons of designating BED as a disorder are well covered in the chapter by Tuschen-Caffier and Schlüssel. The evidence seems to point towards designation as a new eating disorder although whether it causes obesity, or is caused by obesity, or is simply a separate but associated condition is unclear. Because BED has only been relatively recently recognized, as opposed to AN and BN, research into its clinical course and treatment is only now emerging as delineated in the chapters in the section on BED. In some ways it was unfortunate that a substantial body of work on bulimia nervosa preceded the delineation of BED. Hence, treatments for BN were applied without much modification for the treatment of BED. One of the problems associated with doing this was that some of the early steps in treatment research such as using carefully designed control psychotherapies were by-passed in the early work. Hence, it is still unclear whether all treatments are similarly effective in BED, and more importantly whether any are specifically effective for the treatment of BED. A number of studies addressing these issues are now in process and will undoubtedly lead to clarification as to the specificity of treatments such as cognitive-behavioral therapy (CBT) or interpersonal therapy (IPT).

Because the majority of patients with BED are also overweight, the problem of treating both the eating disorder and overweight arises. For the most part, there is little evidence that either CBT or IPT is associated with much in the way of weight loss, although there is some evidence that those who maintain cessation of binge eating do lose weight. This dual problem of an eating disorder accompanied by overweight has been somewhat ignored in the research literature to date, and forms an area for further research. Moreover, because of the short-circuiting of the development of treatment research in BED by applying what was already known for the treatment of BN, we may have overlooked aspects of the psychopathology of BED that may call for different and novel approaches to treatment specifically designed for BED.

Stewart Agras
Stanford, Calif.

Munsch S, Beglinger C (eds): Obesity and Binge Eating Disorder.
Bibl Psychiatr. Basel, Karger, 2005, No 171, pp 1–20

Control of Food Intake

Jean-Pierre Gutzwiller, Christoph Beglinger

Division of Gastroenterology, University Hospital, Basel, Switzerland

A great deal of research interest is directed toward understanding the control of appetite and regulation of metabolism. It seems as if an epidemic of obesity is sweeping the world and type II diabetes is following in its wake. The regulation of energy homeostasis is an area that straddles neurobiology, classical endocrinology and metabolism. It is currently one of the most exciting and rapidly advancing topics in medical research; it is also one of the most frustrating. For even though numerous leaps in scientific understanding have been made, these have not yet been rewarded by any major breakthrough in the practical treatment of human nutritional disorders. Three decades ago, the concept of food intake control was quite simple and consisted of two main centers: (1) The ventromedial hypothalamic nuclei (VMH), perceived as the 'satiety centre'. Stimulation of these nuclei inhibits feeding whereas lesions in this region result in hyperphagia and weight gain [1]. (2) The lateral hypothalamic area (LHA), viewed as a 'feeding centre' whose actions oppose those of the VMH. Electrical stimulation of this region increases food intake [2] while damage here leads to fatal anorexia and wasting [3].

In the past decade, research has identified an increasing number of peptides and other neurotransmitters that are involved in appetite control. Even though much of the research has been carried out on animals, these models have parallels in humans. Metabolism or energy balance is primarily regulated by the central nervous system (CNS), which uses a wide range of humoral and neural signals to sense the metabolic status and control energy intake. Appetite control is dependent on the peripheral physiology and the signals from metabolic processes which are transmitted to the brain. The general mechanism for appetite control involves the intake of food followed by release of peptides from the GI tract, which then sends feedback signals to the brain. These feedback signals pass as hormones through the blood via the arcuate nucleus (ARC) to subcortical brain centers or, through afferent fibers of the vagal nerve via the nucleus tractus solitarius (NTS) into the brainstem.

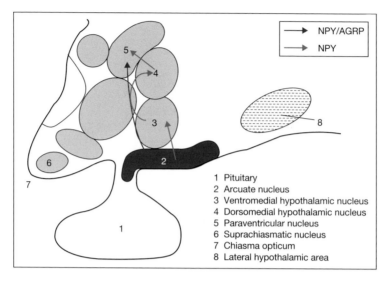

Fig. 1. Intrathalamic signals. Pathways from the arcuate nucleus to the paraventricular nucleus are mediated through neuropeptide Y (NPY) and/or alternatively, through agouti-gene related peptide (AGRP). Pathways from the arcuate nucleus (ARC) to the ventromedial hypothalamic nucleus (VMH), from the VMH to the dorsomedial hypothalamic nucleus (DMH) and from the DMH to the paraventricular nucleus (PVN) are mediated through NPY.

Central Anatomical Sites for Appetite Regulation

Knowledge about this topic has been gleaned from data obtained from experiments in rodents. Some of the lessons learned from lower mammals may also apply to man, although the strength and emphasis of the message may differ between the species. The basic organization of the hypothalamus is illustrated in figure 1.

The ARC lies in the floor of the third ventricle and occupies almost half of the length of the hypothalamus. The ARC contains several functionally discrete populations of neurons. These include one that expresses the orexigenic (appetite-stimulating) neuropeptides, neuropeptide Y (NPY) and agouti-related peptide (AGRP), while another contains pro-opiomelanocortin (POMC) and cocaine- and amphetamine-related transcript (CART) neurons, which are anorexigenic (appetite-inhibiting) [4]. The ARC lies within the mediobasal hypothalamus, where the blood-brain barrier (BBB) is specially modified to render this region easily accessible to circulating hormones, such as leptin, insulin, ghrelin and the glucocorticoids. All these centres are involved in signalling the nutritional state and in regulating appetite.

The ARC has extensive reciprocal connections with other hypothalamic regions that control energy balance, including the paraventricular nuclei (PVN), ventromedial hypothalamic (VMH) and dorsomedial hypothalamic (DMH) nuclei, as well as the lateral hypothalamic area (LHA) (cf. fig. 1).

The PVN, located beside the top of the third ventricle in the anterior hypothalamus, is the site of convergence for many neuronal pathways that regulate energy homeostasis. These include projections from the NPY/AGRP and POMC/CART neurons in the ARC, and from the orexin neurons of the LHA. The PVN also contains neurons that express corticotrophin-releasing factor, an appetite-inhibiting peptide that is released in the ARC and apparently acts to inhibit the NPY neurons.

The large VMH was long considered a 'satiety centre', as mentioned above. Although this hypothesis now appears to be overly simplistic, recent studies have shown that the VMH neurons abundantly contain the long isoform of the leptin receptor (Ob-Rb) [5]. This implicates this region as being an important target for circulating leptin, the adipocyte-derived hormone that acts on the brain to inhibit feeding.

In addition, the VMH is rich in glucose-responsive neurons; these respond to an increase in blood glucose levels and may help to terminate feeding [6]. The VMH has direct connections with the PVN and DMH and through them, may connect indirectly with the LHA.

The diffuse LHA contains separate populations of neurons that express the orexigenic peptides, orexin-A and melanin-concentrating hormone (MCH). NPY terminals are abundant in the LHA where they form synaptic connections with the orexin-A and MCH cell bodies; this region is also rich in the NPY Y5 receptors have been proposed as mediating the appetite-stimulating effects of NPY [7]. The LHA, classically viewed as a 'feeding centre', is rich in glucose-sensitive neurons that are excited by a decrease in the blood glucose concentration, itself a powerful stimulus to feeding.

The DMH, located immediately above the VMH, contains abundant insulin and leptin (Ob-Rb) receptors. ARC NPY/AGRP neurons also terminate here. The DMH has extensive connections with other hypothalamic nuclei. The DMH and the PVN are thought to integrate opposing signals from the VMH and the LHA, effectively acting as a functional unit that initiates, maintains and ultimately terminates feeding [8].

The regulation of energy homeostasis also involves multiple brain regions outside the hypothalamus. The medulla contains the nucleus tractus solitarius (NTS), which receives sensory inputs from the viscera and relays them to the hypothalamus. These visceral signals, carried by sensory (afferent) fibers of the vagus nerve, include gastric distension and portal vein glucose levels, and thus depict the nutritional state as perceived by the gut. Cholecystokinin

(CCK), the intestinal peptide released by the duodenum and involved in meal termination, also sends signals to the NTS via receptors (CCK1) on sensory terminals of the vagal nerve. Taste is another sensory modality conveyed to the NTS.

Central Signals Involved in Satiety Regulation

The hypothalamus contains many different neurotransmitters and peptides – to date, more than 50 have been reported. Many can influence feeding behavior and energy metabolism under experimental conditions in rodents. Most of these neurotransmitters have been identified within the human hypothalamus, but relatively little is known about their neuronal pathways, sites of release or possible functions in humans.

Neuropeptide Y
NPY, a 36-amino acid neurotransmitter belonging to the pancreatic polypeptide family, is one of the most abundant and widely distributed neurotransmitters in the mammalian central nervous system, including man. NPY concentrations are particularly high in the hypothalamus, mostly derived from neurons in the ARC, 90% of which also express AGRP [9]. NPY injected into cerebral ventricles or directly into the PVN, DMH or LHA induces pronounced hyperphagia – indeed, NPY is one of the most potent central appetite stimulants known. Chronic NPY administration induces obesity and it must also be mentioned that overactivity of the ARC NPY neurons is thought to contribute to has been implicated in hyperphagia. The orexigenic action of NPY is thought to be mediated by specific subtypes of NPY receptors, probably Y5, with Y1 likely playing an additional role [10]. ARC NPY neurons become overactive in animals that have lost body weight and fat through energy deficits, such as starvation, lactation, or insulin-deficient diabetes. They also become overactive in rodents with genetic obesity that is due either to leptin receptor defects or to a loss of biologically active leptin (ob/ob mouse). However, NPY does not appear to mediate overeating under all conditions, nor in all forms of obesity. ARC NPY neuronal activity is reduced in rats with dietary obesity induced by voluntary overeating of a palatable diet; the neurons may be inhibited in an attempt to limit overeating and weight gain. Surprisingly, transgenic knockout mice that lack NPY eat and grow normally [11]. However, this does not rule out a role for the NPY system in regulating food intake, but instead highlights the potential for other neuronal systems or transmitters to take over from NPY – indeed, this ability to be overridden is a general caveat when using the knockout approach to explore the control of energy homeostasis. Using NPY knockout mice, it has

been shown that AGRP messenger RNA and immunoreactivity are upregulated with fasting, suggesting that AGRP (also produced by the NPY neurons) may compensate for the lack of NPY in this model [12].

Melanocyte-Stimulating Hormones and Melanocortin Receptors

The melanocortin neurons produce various peptides derived from a common precursor, pro-opio-melanocortin (POMC). POMC is synthesized in specific neurons of the ARC and NTS. Three melanocortin receptor subtypes, MC3-R, MC4-R, and MC5-R, have been located in the brain; both MC3-R and MC4-R are expressed within specific hypothalamic nuclei, including the VMH, DMH and ARC-ME (arcuate nucleus-median eminence) [13, 14]. Both MC3-R and MC4-R probably mediate the hypophagic effects of the melanocortins, but recent studies have assigned MC4-R the principal role. MC4-R knockout mice display obesity [15]. MC3-R knockout mice become obese; adiposity develops despite reduced food intake, apparently because of greater feeding efficiency, while mice lacking both MC3-R and MC4-R demonstrate greater obesity than when MC4-R alone is deficient [16]. Thus, both of these melanocortin receptors probably participate in the regulation of body weight.

The melanocortin system responds to various peripheral signals of nutritional status, notably leptin. Approximately 30% of ARC POMC neurons express the Ob-Rb isoform of the leptin receptor. Intraperitoneal leptin administration increases hypothalamic POMC mRNA levels while conditions associated with decreased leptin (e.g. fasting) or mutations that cause loss of the leptin signal (ob/ob and fa/fa) show decreased POMC mRNA levels [17]. Leptin therefore appears to stimulate POMC neurons, consistent with the observation that both inhibit feeding. There is also evidence that leptin may act on a particular subset of neurons (POMC or NPY/AGRP) that project specifically to MC4-R in the VMH, and so determine an individual rat's susceptibility to dietary-induced obesity [18].

AGRP, expressed in NPY neurons of the ARC, may be regulated more rigorously by an altered metabolic state than by the melanocortins themselves. Changes in AGRP concentrations are observed in dietary-obese and food-restricted animals in the absence of any alterations in α-MSH or POMC [19]. This suggests that AGRP may fine-tune the activity of the melanocortin axis. The melanocortin axis also operates in humans as confirmed by recent observations that rare cases of morbid obesity are associated with specific mutations affecting components of this system [20].

Orexins

Orexin-A and orexin-B are two homologous peptides of 33- and 28-amino acid residues, respectively [21]. Orexins/hypocretins are expressed by specific neurons restricted to the perifornical nuclei and dorsal and lateral areas of the hypothalamus. Orexin neurons also interact with other appetite-regulating neuronal systems, and reciprocal connections between orexin neurons and ARC NPY/AGRP and POMC/CART populations have been identified [22]. Central orexin administration stimulates feeding, and this action gave the peptides their name [Greek orexis: appetite].

It appears that the nutritional conditions under which orexin neurons are activated are very tightly controlled, with decreased plasma glucose and the absence of food from the gut both being required. Acute hypoglycemia activates orexin neurons, but this response is prevented by allowing the animals to eat, suggesting that the presence of food in the gut (e.g. gastric distension) may generate inhibitory signals [24]. Such signals are known to be transmitted via vagal sensory fibers to the NTS, whence important projections ascend to the LHA, the site of the orexin neuron cell bodies (cf. fig. 1). Current evidence indicates that the orexins are involved in the short-term regulation of feeding rather than the long-term control of body weight.

Orexin-A induces acute hyperphagia, particularly during daytime, which can be blocked by specific antagonists. The stimulation of feeding is short-lived: the overall 24-hour intake is not increased after a single injection nor does obesity follow chronic intracerebroventricular administration [23]. Orexin-B has a much weaker effect in stimulating feeding.

Glucose-Sensing Neurons

Glucose is the main metabolic fuel of the brain, and decreases in blood glucose concentration potently stimulate feeding. Specific CNS regions, notably the PVN, VMH, ARC and LHA, as well as the NTS, contain glucose-sensing neurons that detect changes in glucose availability. Glucose-sensing neurons fall into two classes: glucose-responsive neurons (GRN), which increase their firing rate as glucose levels increase; and glucose-sensitive neurons (GSN), which are stimulated by decreases in glucose [25]. It has been postulated that changes in glucose availability are important in the short-term regulation of feeding. A transient, small decrease in blood glucose levels (~0.5 mmol/l) precedes most spontaneous feeding episodes in rats, and giving exogenous glucose at this time can abolish feeding [26]. It has therefore been assumed that GSN and GRN are respectively involved in initiating and terminating feeding in response to changes in glucose levels, but this hypothesis has not been vigorously tested. It is now becoming clear that glucose-sensing neurons are affected by circulating factors other than glucose – for example, leptin and insulin both inhibit the GRN of the VMH [27] as well as interact with other appetite-regulating neuronal systems, such as the orexin pathways [28].

Signal Pathways and Factors from the Gut to the Brain

The gastrointestinal (GI) tract accepts ingested food and processes it, both mechanically and chemically, into small, absorbable units. Thus, carbohydrates are processed in the stomach and small intestine into fatty acids and monosaccharides; lipids are transformed into glycerol and fatty acids; and finally, proteins are cleaved to amino acids. All these digestive end products plus micronutrients, such as vitamins and minerals, become absorbed by the body. The entire process of digestion is coordinated by interactions of the enteric nervous system that innervates the walls of the GI tract. Many gastrointestinal factors are released from specialized endocrine cells into the circulation or serve as neurotransmitters mediating signals from the enteric nervous system. These signals are transmitted from the gut to the brain and become integrated at various centers in the hypothalamus, reflecting the load of nutrients ingested. As a group, these peptides are called satiety signals because most create a sensation of fullness in humans and reduce food intake when administered to humans or animals.

Several criteria must be fulfilled before a hormone or neurotransmitter can be considered a satiety signal. First, the signal must exert a reducing effect on the meal size. Second, it should evoke the opposite effect when it is blocked by a specific receptor antagonist. The knockout experiment is one approach used to follow what happens when the factor under investigation is not present, i.e. it has been 'knocked out'. Third, the reduction in food intake caused by administration of such a 'satiety' signal should not be the consequence of illness or malaise. Fourth, the secretion of an endogenous satiety signal must be induced by ingested food, and the pharmacological profile must be related to the ingestion of meals. However, this condition can only be applied to humoral factors.

Looking at ingestive behavior, most meals are initiated at times that are convenient or habitual and are therefore based more on social or learned factors rather than on adjustments of energy levels within the body. Because of this, the regulation of food intake is evidenced by how much food will be consumed when a meal is eaten [41]. This type of control allows considerable flexibility, such that individuals can adapt their meal patterns to their environment and lifestyle while still maintaining control over the amount of food consumed and integrating this with body fat. The satiety system, as its name implies, determines meal size which is equated with the phenomenon of satiety or fullness.

Cholecystokinin (CCK)

The duodenal peptide, CCK, is the most extensively studied satiety signal. It is secreted from duodenal cells in response to nutrients in the lumen;

the specific nutrients that are most effective in evoking its release vary among the different species. Part of the secreted CCK enters the blood and stimulates the exocrine pancreas and gallbladder to secrete appropriate enzymes into the duodenum, thereby facilitating the digestive process. In 1973, Gibbs et al. [42] administered purified or synthetic CCK to rats before a meal and observed that meal size was reduced in a dose-dependent fashion. Since then, dozens of experiments have documented the ability of exogenous CCK to reduce meal size in numerous species, including humans [43, 44].

The role of the preabsorptive release of CCK in the production of meal-ending satiety has been extensively studied in animals [45, 46]. The effect of CCK on food intake was shown to be an interaction of various factors: Muurahainen and coworkers suggested that a preload of a liquid meal inducing gastric distension together with a concomitant infusion of CCK-8 could reduce food intake in humans. Later, using the CCK1-receptor antagonist, loxiglumide, our group demonstrated that this combined effect was mediated by CCK1-receptors [47]. In another study, we showed that endogenous CCK mediates fat-induced reduction of food intake, and that CCK participates in the interaction of intraduodenal fat with the stomach to regulate food intake in humans, an effect mediated by CCK1-receptors [48]. However, mice with a targeted deletion of the CCK1-receptor have normal body weight, implying either mechanisms to compensate for the lacking CCK1 signalling, or that CCK may not be involved in long-term body weight maintenance in mice. The most popular conceptualization of the mechanism by which CCK works is that when nutrients enter the duodenum and stimulate CCK secretion, some of the CCK acts in a local paracrine manner to stimulate CCK1-receptors on the sensory fibers of the vagus nerves [101]. Other branches of the same vagal sensory nerves carry information from the stomach wall and elsewhere, and thus the same neurons can be sensitive to both CCK and other stimuli, such as gastric distension. This information is then transported to the brain through the nucleus tractus solitarius.

Glugacon-Like Peptide-1 (GLP-1)
The pro-glucagon-derived glucagon-like peptide-1(7–36)amide (GLP-1) is a gastrointestinal hormone that is released in response to food intake from the distal small intestine [49, 50]. Its biological effects include a glucose-dependent insulinotropic effect on the pancreatic B cells and inhibition of gastric emptying. This last effect can be interpreted as being part of the 'ileal break mechanism', an endocrine feedback loop that is activated by nutrients in the ileum [50, 51]. In addition, GLP-1 has been proposed as playing a physiological regulatory role in controlling appetite and energy intake in humans

[52, 53] and in animals [54, 55]. This observation can be extended to patients with obesity and diabetes mellitus type 2 [56, 57]. Recent data suggest that longer term subcutaneous infusions of GLP-1 for 6 weeks even reduces body weight [58]. This study could demonstrate that GLP-1's effect on food intake does not exhibit tachyphylaxis, and also makes the concept suitable for a new treatment approach in patients with diabetes type 2 and weight problems. Thus, long-acting GLP-1 analogues are becoming available for human use [59, 60].

Although it is established that GLP-1 exerts specific functions in the central nervous system [55], the exact mechanisms by which the peptide influences feeding behavior have not yet been completely clarified. The wide distribution of GLP-1 receptors in the area postrema [61–64] implies that central effects may be involved in the reduction of food ingestion following GLP-1 infusion. An additional inhibition of gastrointestinal motility by GLP-1 [65–67] may reduce feelings of hunger and, in turn, increase satiety. It is still incompletely understood how peripherally secreted or injected GLP-1 can evoke central effects as most of the GLP-1 binding sites in the hypothalamic and extrahypothalamic nuclei are separated from the circulation by the blood-brain barrier. It is possible that peripherally injected or secreted GLP-1 could stimulate peripheral vagal afferent nerve fibers that project to central nuclei in the hypothalamus. Another possible mode of action could be transport into the central nervous system via specific carriers or endothelial leaks, making peripheral GLP-1 accessible to central binding sites [68]. It is likely that GLP-1 exerts its effect on the regulation of food intake via a specific interaction with binding sites in certain areas of the central nervous system from where efferent projections are directed to the hypothalamus. Finally, an important observation is the fact that obese subjects have an attenuated postprandial GLP-1 secretion after oral carbohydrate ingestion [69].

Peptide YY$_{3-36}$

Peptide YY$_{3-36}$ (PYY) is synthesized and released from specialized endocrine cells in the gut (L-cells), found primarily in the distal gastrointestinal tract. The same cells synthesize and release GLP-1. In response to the ingestion of nutrients, PYY levels increase within 15 min, peak at 60 min, and remain elevated for up to 6 h [70]. Similar to GLP-1, the initial increase occurs before nutrients have reached the L cells, suggesting a neuronal or endocrine mechanism. The sustained release is thought to be due to the direct effects of the intraluminal gut contents on the L-cells [71]. PYY acts via NPY Y2 (Y2R) receptors as a Y2R-agonist [72]. It was recently demonstrated that peripherally-injected PYY inhibits food intake in mice and human volunteers [73]. Activity of c-Fos was observed in the arcuate nucleus. Peripheral infusion of

PYY in Y2R-deficient mice did not influence food intake, suggesting that PYY acts through Y2R receptors in the arcuate nucleus. The same group observed that PYY levels are low in obesity, indicating PYY's influence in the pathogenesis of this condition [74]. PYY infused into obese patients reduced food intake [74].

Ghrelin

Ghrelin, a recently discovered 28-amino acid peptide, is – in contrast to all factors mentioned above – an orexigenic peptide. Synthesis of ghrelin occurs predominantly in epithelial cells lining the fundus of the stomach. Ghrelin is secreted in a pulsatile manner, similar to leptin. Interestingly, the gherlin receptor was known well before ghrelin was discovered. Cells within the anterior pituitary bear a receptor that, when activated, potently stimulates secretion of growth hormone (GH) – and the receptor was named growth hormone secretagogue receptor (GHS-R). In 1999, the natural ligand for the GHS-R was announced as ghrelin, so named for its ability to provoke growth hormone secretion. Ghrelin receptors are present on the pituitary cells that secrete growth hormone, and have also been identified in the hypothalamus, heart and adipose tissue.

In both rodents and humans, ghrelin functions to increase feelings of hunger through its action on hypothalamic feeding centers. This makes sense with respect to the increased plasma ghrelin concentrations observed during fasting. Several investigators noted that either intracerebroventricular or intraperitoneal ghrelin stimulated food intake as well as GH secretion in rats [75–77], and the orexigenic effect was comparable to that of neuropeptide Y (NPY) [78, 79]. Later experiments in volunteers demonstrated that intravenous ghrelin enhanced appetite and increased food intake [80]. Preprandial ghrelin levels are, on average, 80% higher than postprandial ghrelin concentrations suggesting an important role of the peptide in meal initiation in humans [81]. Interestingly, a diet-induced weight loss is associated with a higher AUC of ghrelin, which is consistent with the hypothesis that ghrelin has a role in the regulation of body weight [82]. In contrast, patients who have undergone gastric bypass show reduced ghrelin levels. This phenomenon might contribute to the degree and duration of weight loss achieved after gastric bypass surgery [82]. The fact that ghrelin levels are decreased by caloric load to the stomach, rather than bygastric distension alone, suggests involvement of gastric chemosensory afferents [75]. After administration of ghrelin, there is an increase in c-Fos mRNA expression in the arcuate nucleus of the hypothalamus [83]. More than 90% of NPY neurons possess GHS-R mRNA [84]. Because of these results and the fact that NPY has orexigenic effects, it was assumed that ghrelin acts via activation of NPY in the arcuate nucleus. Blockade of the gastric vagal afferents by vagotomy and capsaicin abolished ghrelin-induced feeding and activation of NPY neurons, implicating that ghrelin signalling is mediated through the vagus nerve [86]. However, induction of hunger by ghrelin is not solely mediated by NPY. When ghrelin is administered to NPY knockout mice, they still put on weight [75], and there is evidence of increased agouti-related peptide mRNA in the hypothalamus [85].

Role of Adipose Tissue

Recent clinical and experimental data have radically modified the concept of adipose tissue as being solely devoted to energy storage and release. Adipose tissue is critical for maintaining energy balance: it serves both as a storage depot and an endocrine organ. It is likewise actively involved in sensing the nutritional state of the organism through several different signalling pathways. Identification of leptin, a hormone synthesized by adipose tissue, has ushered in the modern view that it is a true endocrine organ.

Leptin
Leptin [Greek leptos: thin] is the product of the ob gene, identified in late 1994 on mouse chromosome 6 [29]. The ob gene is highly conserved among vertebrates. Mouse leptin shares 84% sequence identity to the product of the human ob gene, which lies on chromosome 7q31.3 [30]. Leptin is mainly produced in adipose tissue and secreted into the bloodstream; lower levels of expression are also found in the brown adipose tissue, stomach and placenta of rodents. The expression and secretion of leptin shows circadian variation and is stimulated by insulin and glucocorticoids, which may explain the fall in expression during fasting [31, 32]. Two mutations have been identified in the mouse ob gene; both lead to the ob/ob syndrome of hyperphagia, obesity and diabetes mellitus type 2 [33].

The leptin receptors (OB-R) were first isolated from mouse choroids, and exist as several splice variants that are expressed in various tissues [34]. The isoform that mainly mediates the effect of leptin on body weight, OB-Rb, contains all the intracellular motifs required for efficient activation of the JAK-STAT signal transduction pathway (JAK, Janus Kinases; STAT, Signal Transducer and Activators of Transcription) [35]. OB-Rb is highly abundant in the hypothalamus where it is expressed by the NPY/AGRP and POMC/CART neurons of the ARC, and by MCH and orexin neurons in the LHA. These neurons, and others in sites such as the NTS, appear to mediate some of leptin's central actions, including inhibition of feeding [17].

Leptin circulates at levels proportional to body fat mass in rodents, humans and other mammals [33]. When injected into rodents either systemically or intracerebroventricularly, leptin decreases food intake and increases BAT (brown adipose tissue) activity and whole body energy expenditure, ultimately causing loss of weight and body fat [33]. Circulating leptin can rapidly cross the BBB to enter the mediobasal hypothalamus and may also reach periventricular regions via the cerebrospinal fluid. Leptin inhibits the ARC NPY neurons [36], but NPY-knockout transgenic mice also decrease feeding following leptin administration, indicating that leptin also acts on other neuronal systems [11]. Absence of biologically-active leptin (as in the ob/ob mouse) or failure of the brain to perceive it (the db/db mouse and fa/fa rat) leads to hyperphagia, reduced BAT thermogenic activity and increased fat accumulation.

In humans, under conditions of consistent food intake, the primary determinant of serum leptin is the amount of body fat. Leptin is highly correlated with fat mass in adults, children and newborns. Serum leptin is elevated in obesity and significantly reduced in lipodystrophic states [87–89]. The elevation in serum leptin in obesity appears to result from both increased fat mass and an increased leptin release from larger adipocytes in obese subjects. Leptin gene expression is greater in larger than in smaller adipocytes [90]; in addition, there is a strong correlation between leptin secretion and fat cell volume [91].

Serum leptin is significantly greater in women than in men with equivalent body fat mass [92]. One explanation for this finding is that, compared to men, women have a significantly greater subcutaneous adipose tissue mass relative to omental adipose mass. Studies using adipose tissue obtained from females have demonstrated that, in the same subject, leptin gene expression and leptin production are greater in subcutaneous than in omental adipocytes [93].

Changes in the amount of adipose tissue alter leptin mRNA levels in the adipocyte and the serum concentration of leptin. A decrease in adipose tissue due to weight loss results in a decrease in circulating leptin, whereas an increase in adipose tissue with weight gain significantly increases leptin [94]. Caloric intake influences serum leptin independently of changes in adipose tissue mass. Several in vivo and in vitro studies suggest that the signal linking energy intake and leptin synthesis in the adipocyte is actually glucose and insulin. Serum leptin falls with short-term fasting (24 h) and increases within 4–5 h after renewed feeding. Maintenance of euglycemia prevents the fasting-induced drop in leptin, implicating insulin or glucose as the nutritional signal recognized by the adipocyte for leptin synthesis [95]. In a prolonged study of energy restriction, changes in serum leptin correlated best with changes in glycemia [96].

The diurnal profile of serum leptin is dependent on food intake: shifting a meal by 6 h without changing light or sleep cycles shifts the leptin peak by 5–7 h. The peak in serum leptin concentration occurs at ~2 a.m., and this is the same for lean and obese subjects under normal physiologic conditions. A dependency on day/night activity has also been shown: reversal of this activity shifts the serum peak by 12 h [97].

Insulin

Insulin is another well-characterized adiposity signal; it circulates at levels that parallel fat mass and its concentrations increase after feeding. Insulin has been proposed as a signal for inducing food intake [98]. This hypothesis is supported by studies showing that, in mice eating a high-fat diet, disabling the insulin receptor in the central nervous system enhances their sensitivity to develop obesity. Clinical support for this idea also comes from studies where insulin secretion is blocked by a somatostatin agonist [99]. When children with hypothalamic obesity were treated with a somatostatin agonist, the degree of reduction in weight was related to the reduction in insulin secretion, as seen during an oral glucose tolerance test. In a subset of severely obese adults, monthly injections of a somatostatin agonist suppressed weight gain.

Similar to leptin, insulin can enter specific brain regions. This may occur either by a crossing of the BBB using a specific transport mechanism, such as one involving insulin receptors on the brain microvessels, or by being transported into the cerebrospinal fluid [37]. Insulin receptors are widely expressed in the brain, and include the ARC, PVN, olfactory bulb, choroid plexus and brainstem [38].

There is much evidence that insulin acts as a satiety factor on the brain in a manner similar to leptin. Injections of subhypoglycemic insulin doses into the cerebral ventricles of rats reduces food intake, whereas injecting insulin antibodies into the VMH increases feeding [39]. In addition to decreased leptin levels, decreases in peripheral insulin may contribute to NPY neuronal hyperactivity and thus increase hunger feelings. It must be mentioned that the intracellular signalling pathways for insulin and leptin might well be the same [40]. Finally, evidence that glucose and insulin regulate leptin production has been obtained with euglycemic-hyperinsulinemic clamp techniques: serum leptin is elevated by the end of prolonged (9 h) euglycemic-hyperinsulinemic clamps at physiologic insulin concentrations [100]. The pathways described in the chapter by Langhans and Geary (this volume) are summarized in figure 2.

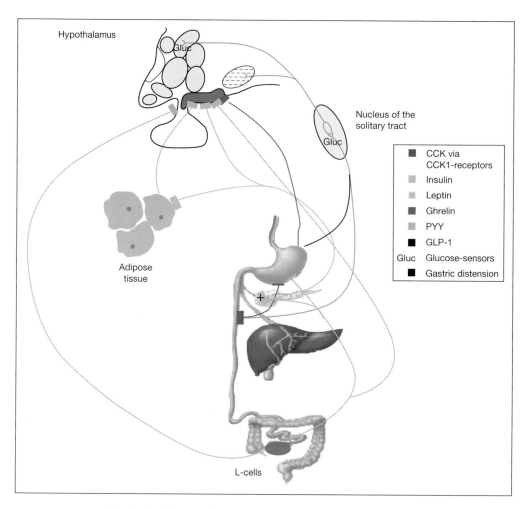

Fig. 2. Peripheral satiety signals. This schematic presentation depicts the concept of peripheral satiety signals and their connection to the brain. Fat induced satiety signals are mediated through CCK via peripheral CCK1-receptors. CCK also inhibits gastric emptying, insulin interacts with leptin on fat cells in the adipose tissue. In addition, it induces satiety through the arcuate nucleus (ARC). Leptin is released by adipose tissue and modulates satiety in different hypothalamic centers., ghrelin is released from the stomach (fundus cells) and induces hunger feelings via the ARC. PYY, which is colocalized with GLP-1 in the L-cells in the distal ileum, induces satiety; PYY is part of a mechanism called the 'ileal brake'. GLP-1 increases insulin secretion and insulin sensitivity in the pancreatic β-cells. In addition, it inhibits gastric emptying and induces satiety. It is not clear whether this occurs through the vagus and nucleus of the solitary tract or through the ARC. Glucose sensors are located in the NTS and in the paraventricular nucleus. A drop in glucose induces hunger. Gastric distension amplifies satiety signals via the NTS.

Conclusion

The concept of food intake control has become more complex as our understanding of the subject has increased. Decades ago, the generally-accepted theory proposed that there was a central controller with two hypothalamic centers, one for hunger and one for satiety. Research has shown that the control of food intake is the complex result of an integration of humoral and neural signals among peripheral tissues, such as the gastrointestinal tract and the adipose tissue, and the brain. Peripheral tissues send feedback signals to the brain which act as hormones travelling through the blood via the arcuate nucleus, or as neurotransmitters via the vagal nerve and the nucleus tractus solitarius.

Neuropeptides from the GI tract, such as cholecystokinin, glucagon-like peptide-1, peptide YY and ghrelin are important biological messengers that carry information to the brain about the digestive state of ingested food in the bowel lumen.

Adipose tissue signals, such as those from leptin and insulin which relay information to the brain, clearly demonstrate the importance of body fat tissue in food intake control. All these signals become integrated into a complex system in different, interconnected hypothalamic centers. The arcuate nucleus is a very important centre in the floor of the third ventricle occupying almost half of the length of the hypothalamus and belonging to the blood brain barrier. Feedback signals are integrated and distributed to other hypothalamic centers, such as the paraventricular nuclei, ventromedial hypothalamic and dorsomedial hypothalamic nuclei, and the lateral hypothalamic area as well. Central neurotransmitters, such as neuropeptide Y, agouti-gene related peptide, the pro-opiomelanocortin system and the orexins mediate these signals between the different hypothalamic centers. These mechanisms are influenced by the glucose concentration, which is continuously measured by glucose-sensing neurons in the hypothalamus.

The complexity of this regulation system demonstrates the importance of a balance in genetic, social, behavioral and environmental factors that all contribute to influencing the control of food intake.

Acknowledgements

Supported by grants from the Swiss National Science Foundation (No. 3200–065588.01/1) and by a grant from the European Commission, Moebius-IST 1999–1159. We would like to express our special thanks to Kathleen Bucher for editing the manuscript.

References

1   Stellar E: The physiology of motivation. Psychol Rev 1954;61:5–22.
2   Steinbaum EA, Miller NE: Obesity from eating elicited by daily stimulation of hypothalamus. Am J Physiol 1965;208:1–5.
3   Winn P, Robbins TW: Comparative effects of infusions of 6-hydroxydopamine into nucleus accumbens and anterolateral hypothalamus induced by 6-hydroxydopamine on the response to dopamine agonists, body weight, locomotor activity and measures of exploration in the rat. Neuropharmacology 1985;24:25–31.
4   Elias CF, Lee C, Kelly J, Aschkenasi C, Ahima RS, Couceyro PR, Kuhar MJ, Saper CB, Elmquist JK: Leptin activates hypothalamic CART neurones projecting to the spinal cord. Neuron 1998; 21:1375–1385.
5   Funahashi H, Yada T, Muroya S, Takigawa M, Ryushi T, Horie S, Nakai Y, Shioda S: The effect of leptin on feeding-regulating neurons in the rat hypothalamus. Neurosci Lett 1999;264:117–120.
6   Oomura Y, Ono T, Ooyama H, Wagner MJ: Glucose and osmosensitive neurons of the rat hypothalamus. Nature 1969;222:282–284.
7   Hu Y, Bloomquist BT, Cornfield LJ, DeCarr LB, Flores-Riveros JR, Friedman L, Jiang P, Lewis-Higgins L, Sadlowski Y, Schaefer J, Velazquez N, McCaleb ML: Identification of a novel hypothalamic neuropeptide Y receptor associated with feeding behavior. J Biol Chem 1996;271: 26315–26319.
8   Christophe J: Is there appetite after GLP-1 and PACAP? Ann N Y Acad Sci 1998;865:323–335.
9   Allen YS, Adrian TE, Allen JM, Tatemoto K, Crow TJ, Bloom SR, Polak JM: Neuropeptide Y distribution in rat brain. Science 1983;221:877–879.
10 Yokosuka M, Dube MG, Kalra PS, Kalra SP: The mPVN mediates blockade of NPY-induced feeding by a Y5 receptor antagonist: a c-FOS analysis. Peptides 2001;22:507–514.
11 Erickson JC, Clegg KE, Palmiter RD: Sensitivity to leptin and susceptibility to seizures of mice lacking neuropeptide Y. Nature 1996;381:415–418.
12 Marsh DJ, Miura Y, Yagaloff KA, Schwartz MW, Barsh GS, Palmiter RD: Effects of neuropeptide Y deficiency on hypothalamic agouti-gene related protein expression and responsiveness to melanocortin analogues. Brain Res 1999;848:66–77.
13 Roselli-Rehfuss L, Mountjoy KG, Robbins LS, et al: Identification of a receptor for γ melanotropin and other proopiomelanocortin peptides in the hypothalamus and limbic system. Proc Natl Acad Sci USA 1993;90:8856–8860.
14 Harrold JA, Widdowson PS, Williams G: Altered energy balance causes selective changes in melanocortin-4 (MC4-R) but not melanocortin-3 (MC3-R) receptors in specific hypothalamic regions: Further evidence that MC4-R activation is a physiological inhibitor of feeding. Diabetes 1999;48:267–271.
15 Huszar D, Lynch CA, Fairchild-Huntress V, et al: Targeted disruption of the melanocortin-4 receptor results in obesity in mice. Cell 1997;88:131–141.
16 Chen AS, Marsh DJ, Trumbauer ME, et al: Inactivation of the mouse melanocortin-4 receptor results in increased fat mass and reduced lean body mass. Nature 2000;26:97–102.
17 Cheung CC, Clifton DK, Steiner RA: Propiomelanocortin neurons are direct targets for leptin in the hypothalamus. Endocrinology 1997;138:4489–4492.
18 Harrold JA, Williams G, Widdowson PS: Early leptin response to palatable diet predicts dietary obesity in rats: Key role of melanocortin-4 receptors in the ventromedial hypothalamic nucleus. J Neurochem 2000;74:1224–1228.
19 Harrold JA, Williams G, Widdowson PS: Changes in hypothalamic agouti-related peptide (AGRP) but not α-MSH or pro-opiomelanocortin concentrations in dietary-obese and food restricted rats. Biochem Biophys Res Commun 1999;258:574–577.
20 Yeo GSH, Farooqi S. Aminian S, Halsall DJ, Stanhope RG, O'Rahilly S: A frameshift mutation in MC4-R associated with dominantly inherited human obesity. Nat Genet 1998;20:111–112.
21 Sakurai T, Amemiya A, Ashii M, et al: Orexins and orexin receptors – A family of hypothalamic neuropeptides and G protein coupled receptors that regulate feeding behavior. Cell 1998;92: 573–585.

22 Elias CF, Saper CB, Maratos-Flier E, et al: Chemically defined projections linking the mediobasal hypothalamus and the lateral hypothalamic area. J Comp Neurol 1998;402:442–459.

23 Yamanaka A, Sakurai T, Katsumoto T, Yanagisawa M, Goto K: Chronic intracerebroventricular administrations of orexin-A to rats increased food intake in daytime, but has no effect on body weight. Brain Res 1999;849:248–252.

24 Cai XJ, Evans ML, Lister CA, et al: Hypoglycaemia activates orexin neurons and selectively increases hypothalamic orexin B levels: Responses inhibited by feeding and possibly mediated by the nucleus of the solitary tract. Diabetes 2000;50:105–112.

25 Oomura Y, Ono T. Ooyama H, Wayner MJ: Glucose and osmosensitive neurons of the rat hypothalamus. Nature 1969;222:282–284.

26 Smith FJ, Campfield LA: Meal initiation occurs after experimental induction of transient declines in blood glucose. Am J Physiol 1993;265:R1423–R1429.

27 Spanswick D, Smith MA, Mirshamsi S, Routh VH, Ashford ML: Insulin activates ATP-sensitive K^+ channels in hypothalamic neurons of lean, but not obese rats. Nat Neurosci 2000;3: 757–758.

28 Liu XH, Morris R, Spiller D, White M, Williams G: Orexin A preferentially excites glucose-sensitive neurons in the lateral hypothalamus of the rat in vitro. Diabetes 2001;50:2431–2437.

29 Zhang Y, Proenca R, Maffei M, Barone M, Leopold L, Friedman JM: Positional cloning of the mouse obese gene and its human homologue. Nature 1994;372:425–432.

30 Isse N, Ogawa Y, Tamura N, et al: Structural organization and chromosomal assignment of the human obese gene. J Biol Chem 1995;270:27728–32773.

31 Slieker LJ, Sloop KW, Surface PL, et al: Regulation of expression of ob mRNA and protein by glucocorticoids and cAMP. J Biol Chem 1996;27:5301–5304.

32 Bing C, Frankish HM, Pickavance L, et al: Hyperphagia induced by chronic cold exposure is accompanied by decreased plasma leptin levels but is independent of hypothalamic neuropeptide Y. Am J Physiol 1998;274:R62–R68.

33 Friedman JF, Halaas J: Leptin and the regulation of body weight in mammals. Nature 1998;395: 763–770.

34 Tartaglia LA: The leptin receptor. J Biol Chem 1997;272:6093–6096.

35 Bjorbaek C, Uotani S, da Silva B, Flier JS: Divergent signaling capacities of the long and short isoforms of the leptin receptor. J Biol Chem 1997;272:32686–32695.

36 Stephens TW, Basinski M, Bristow PK, et al: The role of neuropeptide Y in the antiobesity action of the obese gene product. Nature 1995;377:530–532.

37 Baura G, et al: Saturable transport of insulin from plasma into the central nervous system of dogs in vivo: A mechanism for regulated insulin delivery to the brain. J Clin Invest 1993;92:1824–1830.

38 Baskin DG, et al: Insulin and leptin: Dual adiposity signals to the brain for the regulation of food intake and body weight. Brain Res 1999;848:114–123.

39 Schwartz MW, Figlewicz DP, Baskin DG, Woods SC, Porte DJ: Insulin in the brain: A hormonal regulator of energy balance. Endocr Rev 1992;13;387–414.

40 Kellerer M, Lammers R, Fritsche A, et al: Insulin inhibits leptin receptor signalling in HEK293 cells at the level of the janus kinase-2: A potential mechanism for hyperinsulinaemia-associated leptin resistance. Diabetologia 2001;44:1125–1132.

41 Woods SC, Schwartz MW, Baskin DG, Seeley RJ: Food intake and the regulation of body weight. Annu Rev Psychol 2000;51:255–277.

42 Gibbs J, Young RC, Smith GP: Cholecystokinin decreases food intake in rats. J Comp Physiol Psychol 1973;84:488–495.

43 Kissileff HR, Pi-Sunyer FX, Thornton J, Smith GP: Cholecystokinin decreases food intake in man. Am J Clin Nutr 1981;34:154–160.

44 Lieverse RJ, Jansen JB, Masclee AM, Lamers CB: Satiety effects of cholecystokinin in humans. Gastroenterology 1994;106:1451–1454.

45 Gregory PC, McFadyen M, Rayner DV: Duodenal infusion of fat, cholecystokinin secretion and satiety in the pig. Physiol Behav 1989;45:1021–1024.

46 Moran TH and McHugh PR: Gastric and nongastric mechanisms for satiety action of cholecystokinin. Am J Physiol 1988;254:R628–R632.

47   Gutzwiller JP, Drewe J, Ketterer S, Hildebrand P, Krautheim A, Beglinger C: Interaction between CCK and a preload on reduction of food intake is mediated by CCK-A receptors in humans. Am J Physiol 2000;279:R189–R195.

48   Matzinger D, Gutzwiller JP, Drewe J, Orban A, Engel R, D'Amato M, Rovati L, Beglinger C: Inhibition of food intake in response to intestinal lipid is mediated by cholexystokinin in humans. Am J Physiol 1999;277:R1718–R1724.

49   Drucker DJ: Glucagon-like peptide. Diabetes 1998;47:159–169.

50   Holst JJ: Enteroglucagon. Annu Rev Physiol 1997;59:257–271.

51   Layer P, Holst JJ, Grandt D, Goebell H: Ileal release of glucagons-like peptide-1 (GLP-1). Association with inhibition of gastric acid secretion in humans. Dig Dis Sci 1995;40:1074–1082.

52   Flint A, Raben A, Astrup A, Holst JJ: Glucagon-like peptide 1 promotes satiety and suppresses energy intake in humans. J Clin Invest 1998;101:515–520.

53   Gutzwiller JP, Goeke B, Drewe J, Hildebrand P, Ketterer S, Handschin D, Winterhalder R, Conen D, Beglinger C: Glucagon-like peptide-1: A potent regulator of food intake in humans. Gut 1999;44:81–86.

54   Tang-Christensen M, Larsen PJ, Goeke R, Fink-Jensen A, Jessop DS, Moller M, Sheikh SP: Central administration of GLP-1(7–36) amide inhibits food and water intake in rats. Am J Physiol 1996;40:R848–R856.

55   Turton MD, O'Shea D, Gunn I, Beak SA, Edwards CM, Meeran K, Choi SJ, Taylor GM, Heath MM, Lambert PD, Wilding JP, Smith DM, Ghatei MA, Herbert J, Bloom S: A role for glucagons-like peptide-1 in the central regulation of feeding. Nature 1996;379:69–72.

56   Flint A, Raben A, Ersboll AK, Holst JJ, Astrup A: The effect of physiological levels of glucagons-like peptide-1 on appetite, gastric emptying, energy and substrate metabolism in obesity. Int J Obes Relat Metab Disord 2001;25:781–792.

57   Gutzwiller JP, Drewe J, Goeke B, Schmidt H, Rohrer B, Lareida J, Beglinger C: Glucagon-like peptide-1 promotes satiety and reduces food intake in patients with diabetes mellitus type 2. Am J Physiol 1999;276:R1541-R1544.

58   Zander M, Madsbad S, Madsen JL, Holst JJ: Effect of 6-week course of glucagon-like peptide 1 on gycaemic control, insulin sensitivity and beta-cell function in type 2 diabetes: A parallel-group study. Lancet 2002;359:824–830.

59   Egan JM, Clocquet AR, Elahi D: The insulinotropic effect of acute exendin-4 administered to humans: Comparison of nondiabetic state to type 2 diabetes. J Clin Endocrinol Metab 2002;87:1282–1290.

60   Chang AM, Jakobsen G, Sturis J, Smith JM, Bloem CJ, An B, Galecki A, Halter JB: The GLP-1 derivative NN2211 restores beta-cell sensitivity to glucose in type 2 diabetic patients after a single dose. Diabetes 2003;52:1786–1791.

61   Shimizu I, Hirota M, Ohboshi C, Shima K: Identification and localization of glucagon-like peptide-1 and its receptor in rat brain. Endocrinology 1987;121:1076–1082.

62   Drucker DJ, Asa S: Glucagon gene expression in vertebrate brain. J Biol Chem 1988;263; 13475–13478.

63   Kanse SM, Kreymann B, Ghatei MA, Bloom SR: Identification and characterization of glucagon-like peptide-1 7–36 amide-binding sites in the rat brain and lung. FEBS Lett 1988;241:209–212.

64   Shughrue PJ, Lane MV, Merchenthaler I: Glucagon-like peptide-1 receptor (GLP1-R) mRNA in the rat hypothalamus. Endocrinology 1996;137:5159–5162.

65   Wettergren A, Wojdemann M, Meisner S, Stadil F, Holst JJ: The inhibitory effect of glucagon-like peptide-1 (GLP-1) 7–36 amide on gastric acid secretion in humans depends on an intact vagal innervation. Gut 1997;40:597–601.

66   Nauck MA, Niedereichholz U, Ettler R, Holst JJ, Orskov C, Ritzel R, Schmiegel WH: Glucagon-like peptide 1 inhibition of gastric emptying outweighs its insulinotropic effects in healthy humans. Am J Physiol 1997;273:E981–E988.

67   Schirra J, Kurwert P, Wank U, Leicht P, Arnold R, Goeke B, Katschinski M: Differential effects of subcutaneous GLP-1 on gastric emptying, antroduodenal motility, and pancreatic function in men. Proc Assoc Am Physicians 1997;109:84–97.

68   Orskov C, Poulsen SS, Møller M, Holst JJ: Glucagon-like peptide-1 receptors in the subfornical organ and the area postrema are accessible to circulating glucagon-like peptide 1. Diabetes 1996;45:832–835.

69   Ranganath LR, Beety LM, Morgan LM, Wright JW, Howland R, Marks V: Attenuated GLP-1 secretion in obesity: Cause or consequence? Gut 1996;38:916–919.

70   Adrian TE, Ferri GL, Bacarese-Hamilton AJ, Fuessl HS, Polak JM, Bloom SR: Human distribution and release of a putative new gut hormone, peptide YY. Gastroenterology 1985;89:1070–1077.

71   Imamura M: Effects of surgical manipulation of the intestine on peptide YY and its physiology. Peptides 2002;23:403–407.

72   Keire DA, et al: Primary structures of PYY, [Pro34] PYY and PYY-(3–36) confer different conformations and receptor selectivity. Am J Physiol 2000;279:G126–G131.

73   Batterham RL, Cowley MA, Small CJ, Herzog H, Cohen MA, Dakin CL, Wren AM, Brynes AE, Low MJ, Ghatei MA, Cone RD, Bloom SR: Gut hormone PYY_{3-36} physiologically inhibits food intake. Nature 2002;418:650–654.

74   Batterham RL, Cohen MA, Ellis SM, Le Roux CW, Withers DJ, Frost GS, Ghatei MA, Bloom SR: Inhibition of food intake in obese subjects by peptide YY_{3-36}. N Engl J Med 2003;349:941–948.

75   Tschop M, Smiley DL, Heiman ML: Ghrelin induces adiposity in rodents. Nature 2000;407:908–913.

76   Wren AM, Small CJ, Ward HL, Murphy KG, Dakin CL, Taheri S, Kennedy AR, Roberts GH, Morgan DG, Ghatei MA, Bloom SR: The novel hypothalamic peptide ghrelin stimulates food intake and growth hormone secretion. Endocrinology 2000;141:4325–4328.

77   Nakazato M, Murakami N, Date Y, Kojima M, Matsuo H, Kangawa K, Matsukura S: A role for ghrelin in the central regulation of feeding. Nature 2001;409:194–198.

78   Asakawa A, Inui A, Kaga T, Yuzuriha H, Nagata T, Ueno N, Makino S, Fujimiya M, Niijima A, Fujino MA, Kasuga M: Ghrelin is an appetite-stimulatory signal from stomach with structural resemblance to motilin. Gastroenterology 2001;120:337–345.

79   Stanley BG, Kyrkouli SE, Lampert S, Leibowitz SF: Neuropeptide Y chronically injected into the hypothalamus: A powerful neurochemical inducer of hyperhphagia and obesity. Peptides 1986;7: 1189–1192.

80   Wren AM, Seal LJ, Cohen MA, Brynes AE, Forst GS, Murphy KG, Dhillo WS, Ghatei MA, Bloom SR: Ghrelin enhances appetite and increases food intake in humans. J Clin Endocrinol Metab 2001;86:5992.

81   Cummings DE, Purnell JQ, Frayo RS, Schmidova K, Wisse BE, Weigle DS: A preprandial rise in plasma ghrelin levels suggests a role in meal initiation in humans. Diabetes 2001;50:1714–1719.

82   Cummings DE, Weigle DS, Frayo RS, Breen PA, Ma MK, Dellinger EP, Purnell JQ: Plasma ghrelin levels after diet-induced weight loss or gastric bypass surgery. N Engl J Med 2002;346: 1623–1630.

83   Hewson AK, Dickson SL: Systemic administration of ghrelin induces Fos and Egr-1 proteins in the hypothalamic arcuate nucleus of fasted and fed rats. J Neuroendocrinol 2000;12: 1047–1049.

84   Willesen MG, Kristensen P, Romer J: Co-localization of growth hormone secretagogue receptor and NPY mRNA in the arcuate nucleus of the rat. Neuroendocrinology 1999;70:306–316.

85   Tschop M, Statnick MA, Suter TM, Heiman ML: GH-releasing peptide-2 increases fat mass in mice lacking NPY: Indication for a crucial mediating role of hypothalamic agouti-related protein. Endocrinology 2002;143:558–568.

86   Date Y, Murakami N, Toshinai K, Matsukura S, Niijima A, Matsuo H, Kangawa K, Nakazato M: The role of the gastric afferent vagal nerve in ghrelin-induced feeding and growth hormone secretion in rats. Gastroenterology 2002;123:1120–1128.

87   Maffei M, Halaas J, Ravussin E, Pratley RE, Lee GH, Zhang Y, Fei H, Kim S, Lallone R, Ranganathan S, Kern PA, Friedman JM: Leptin levels in human and rodents: Measurement of plasma leptin and ob RNA in obese and weight-reduced subjects. Nat Med 1995;1:1155–1161.

88   Garcia-Mayor RV, Andrade MA, Rios M, Lage M, Dieguez C, Casanueva FF: Serum leptin levels in normal children: Relationship to age, gender, body mass index, pituitary-gonadal hormones and pubertal stage. J Clin Endocrinol Metab 1997;82:2849–2855.

89   Schubring C, Kiess W, Englaro P, Rascher W, Dotsch J, Hanitsch S, Attanasio A, Blum WF: Levels of leptin in maternal serum, amniotic fluid, and arterial and venous cord blood: Relation to neonatal and placental weight. J Clin Endocrinol Metab 1997;82:1480–1483.

90   Hamilton BS, Paglia D, Kwan AYM, Deitel M: Increased obese mRNA expression in omental fat cells from massively obese humans. Nat Med 1995;1:953–956.

91 Lonnqvist F, Nordfors L, Jansson M, Thorne A, Schalling M, Arner P: Leptin secretion from adipose tissue of women: Relationship to plasma levels and gene expression. J Clin Invest 1997;99:2398–2404.

92 Rosenbaum M, Leibel RL: Role of gonadal steroids in the sexual dimorphisms in body composition and circulating concentrations of leptin. J Clin Endocrinol Metab 1996;81:3424–3427.

93 Van Harmelen V, Reynisdottir S, Eriksson P, Thorne A, Hoffstedt J, Lonnqvist F, Arner P: Leptin secretion from subcutaneous and visceral adipose tissue of women. Diabetes 198;47:913–917.

94 Caro JF, Sinha MK, Kolaczynski JW, Zhang PL, Considine RV: Leptin: The tale of an obesity gene. Diabetes 1996;45:1455–1462.

95 Boden G, Chen X, Mozzoli M, Ryan I: Effect of fasting on serum leptin in normal human subjects. J Clin Endocrinol Metab 1996;81:3419–3423.

96 Wisse BE, Campfield LA, Marliss EB, Morais JA, Tenenbaum R, Gougeon R: Effect of prolonged moderate and severe energy restriction and refeeding on plasma leptin concentrations in obese women. Am J Clin Nutr 1999;70:321–330.

97 Schoeller DA, Cella LK, Sinha MK, Caro JF: Entrainment of the diurnal rhythm of plasma leptin to meal timing. J Clin Invest 1997;100:1882–1887.

98 Schwartz MW, Woods SC, Porte D, Seeley RJ, Baskin DG: Central nervous system control of food intake. Nature 2000;404:661–671.

99 Lustig RH, Rose SR, Burgben GA, Velasquez-Mieyer P, Broome DC, Smith K, Li H, Hudson MM, Heideman RL, Kun LE: Hypothalamic obesity caused by cranial insult in children: Altered glucose and insulin dynamics and reversal by a somatostatin agonist. J Pediatr 1999;135:162–168.

100 Utriainen T, Malmstrom R, Makimattila S, Yki-Jarvinen H: Supraphysiological hyperinsulinemia increases plasma leptin concentrations after 4 h in normal subjects. Diabetes 1996;45:1364–1366.

101 Moran TH, Baldessarini AR, Salorio CF, Lowery T, Schwartz GJ: Vagal afferent and efferent contributions to the inhibition of food intake by cholecystokinin. Am J Physiol 1997;272:R1245–R1251.

Prof. Dr. med. Ch. Beglinger
Abteilung für Gastroenterologie, Universität Basel
Petersgraben 4, CH–4031 Basel (Switzerland)
Tel. +41 61 265 25 25, Fax +41 61 265 53 52, E-Mail beglinger@tmr.ch

Munsch S, Beglinger C (eds): Obesity and Binge Eating Disorder.
Bibl Psychiatr. Basel, Karger, 2005, No 171, pp 21–40

··························

Regulation of Body Weight

Wolfgang Langhans, Nori Geary

Physiology and Animal Husbandry, Institute of Animal Sciences,
Swiss Federal Institute of Technology (ETH), Zürich, Switzerland

Is Body Weight Regulated?

The prevalence of obesity and obesity-related disorders increases at an alarming rate, in particular in children and adolescents. As a result, obesity may soon overtake smoking as the single most important cause of death in industrialized countries. Although these frightening developments appear to suggest otherwise, body weight in adult individuals in many respects appears to be actively and accurately regulated. This is shown, for example, by calculations indicating that an error in the control system of less than 1% could lead to much larger rates of body weight gain than we are actually experiencing.

In line with this efficient weight maintenance, experimental manipulations of body weight in adult individuals are readily compensated for by changes in energy intake and energy expenditure [1–4], suggesting that both sides of the energy balance equation are involved in this control. Recent evidence in fact indicates that similar anabolic and catabolic neuropeptidergic pathways either produce hunger and decrease energy expenditure at times when endogenous fuels are in short supply, or inhibit feeding and increase energy expenditure in conditions of a surplus of endogenous energy. With all other things being equal, body weight changes in adult individuals are mainly due to fluctuations in body fat, which is therefore the most plausible variable to be regulated. This concept of 'lipostasis' was proposed by Kennedy [5] about 50 years ago. At the core of this concept is the assumption that a circulating factor whose plasma level reflects the size of the fat stores controls food intake and energy expenditure to keep body fat and, hence, body weight stable [5]. The results of numerous cross-perfusion and parabiosis studies confirm this concept of a humoral signal [1, 6, 7].

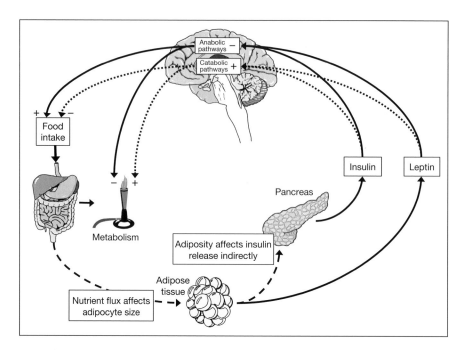

Fig. 1. Leptin and insulin activate catabolic and inhibit anabolic hypothalamic neuropeptide systems that control energy intake and metabolism. The level of adiposity and/or the balance between inflow and outflow of energy in adipocytes determines the release of leptin from adipocytes. Adiposity influences insulin release from the pancreas. Both hormones act in the hypothalamus to produce compensatory ingestive and metabolic responses. See text for further details.

Leptin as a Lipostatic Signal

The discovery of the adipose tissue hormone leptin [8] and its receptor [9] has triggered a tremendous increase in our understanding of the molecular and physiologic pathways of body weight control. Leptin fulfills most of the theoretical predictions for a lipostatic signal phrased by Kennedy [5] (fig. 1). It is expressed in adipose tissue, secreted into the blood in relation to body adiposity [10, 11], binds to receptors in several sites [12–14], and is lowered by fasting or weight loss [11]. Leptin also acts directly on the brain to inhibit eating and to stimulate energy expenditure in genetically obese and normal rodents [15–17], although the physiological status of this remains controversial [18]. The role of leptin in the control of energy balance may be more dynamic than proposed by the original lipostatic hypothesis. Thus, under- or overeating can cause unexpectedly large changes in plasma leptin within 1 or 2 days, i.e. well before any significant weight gain or loss occurs [19, 20]. These findings suggest that the daily flux of energy substrates in and out of the adipocyte may partially control leptin synthesis and release. In addition to acting as a long-term lipostatic signal, leptin may therefore correct day(s)-to-day(s) changes in energy intake and fine-tune it with energy expenditure at normal body weight.

Laboratory animal models of obesity with monogenetic defects in the leptin system, such as the ob/ob mouse and the db/db mouse, provided the basis for the discovery of leptin and have contributed substantially to our understanding of the role of leptin in body weight control. It is clear, however, that, with a few notable exceptions [21, 22], human obesity is not due to single gene mutations. The genetic contribution to the current obesity epidemic merely reflects the fact that evolution has not prepared us for our current environment, with its lack of physical activity and constant abundance of attractive, energy dense food.

In addition to its role in control of energy balance, leptin has been shown to link body weight control to reproductive [23, 24] and immune functions [25] as well as metabolism [26–28]. Leptin has pronounced metabolic effects in the periphery that are not centrally mediated and that appear to contribute to its role in control of body weight [26]. Thus, leptin was recently found to specifically repress RNA levels and enzymatic activity of hepatic stearoyl-CoA desaturase-1 (SCD-1), which catalyzes the biosynthesis of monounsaturated fatty acids [26]. This is interesting because mice genetically deficient in SCD-1 are hypermetabolic and lean. Even ob/ob mice with mutations in SCD-1 were less obese than ob/ob control mice and had markedly increased energy expenditure [26]. Together, these findings suggest that downregulation of SCD-1 contributes to leptin's effect on body weight.

Central Neuropeptide Pathways of Leptin Action

The central processing of the leptin signal is based on changes in the balance of a number of anabolic (e.g. Agouti-related peptide (AgrP), neuropeptide Y (NPY)) and catabolic (e.g. α-melanocyte-stimulating hormone (α-MSH) and cocaine- and amphetamine-regulated transcript (CART)) neuropeptides (fig. 2). The balance among these neuropeptides determines the behavioral and autonomic output that controls eating behavior and metabolism. Leptin controls the expression of these neuropeptides through the long (active) form of the leptin receptor [29–31]. Specific transgenic deletion of the long form of the leptin receptor in the brain leads to obesity [32], indicating that the central effects are an essential component of leptin's effect on body weight.

A group of hypothalamic neurons originating in the arcuate nucleus (ARC) and projecting to the paraventricular nucleus (PVN) and the lateral hypothalamic

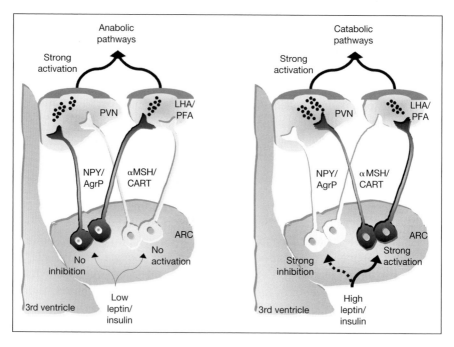

Fig. 2. Activation and inhibition of intrahypothalamic catabolic and anabolic neuro-peptide systems by leptin and insulin. See text for further details. AgrP = Agouti-related peptide, ARC = arcuate nucleus; CART = cocaine- and amphetamine-regulated transcript; LHA = lateral hypothalamic area; αMSH = α-melanocyte-stimulating hormone; NPY = neuropeptide Y; PFA = perifornical area; PVN = paraventricular nucleus.

area (LHA) express NPY and AgrP [33] (fig. 2). NPY has long been known to potently stimulate hunger and reduce energy expenditure when administered into the cerebral ventricles. The peptide AgrP is an endogenous antagonist of melanocortin receptors. A genetic lack of AgrP in mice is accompanied by yellow fur due to the unopposed activation of peripheral melanocortin-1 (MC-1) receptors. Central administration of AgrP in rats induces a longer lasting stimulatory effect on food intake than NPY, which is presumably due to a blockade of central MC-3 and MC-4 receptors [31]. The NPY and AgrP neurons in the ARC possess leptin receptors, and part of the inhibitory effect of leptin on food intake and of its hypermetabolic effect appears to be due to an inhibition of these NPY- and AgrP neurons [31]. Consequently, deletion of the leptin receptor in the brain is accompanied by increased hypothalamic levels of NPY and AgrP [32].

Leptin activates another group of ARC neurons that also expresses two peptides, namely CART and pro-opiomelanocortin (POMC), and/or the POMC-derived α-melanocyte-stimulating hormone (αMSH) [34] (fig. 2). These neurons also project to the PVN and the LHA, and their activation profoundly inhibits eating. The inhibitory effect of POMC/αMSH is mediated by MC-3 and MC-4 receptors on the target cells. The massive obesity observed in humans with genetic defects in the synthesis or action of POMC and its derivatives demonstrates the importance of the POMC-system for the maintenance of energy balance [e.g. 22]. CART was originally identified as a peptide whose transcription is stimulated by cocaine and amphetamine. Yet, CART has also a potent inhibitory effect on food intake, which appears to be recruited by leptin. CART mRNA and peptide are found in several hypothalamic sites [29], and leptin induces c-Fos and CART expression in many of these neurons [35]. ICV CART application reduces, and application of CART antibodies stimulates, food intake in laboratory animals [35]. CART cell bodies and fibers were also found in the human hypothalamus [29], suggesting that CART may also play a role in the control of energy homeostasis in humans.

Downstream of the NPY/AgrP and POMC/CART neurons are presumably several other anabolic and catabolic neurochemicals [29–31], such as melanin concentrating hormone (MCH, anabolic) [36], endogenous opioids [37] (mainly anabolic), the corticotrophin-releasing factor (CRF, catabolic), and others. MCH is a cyclic 19 amino acid peptide, and its role in the control of food intake has been revealed only recently [38]. Through these neuropeptidergic pathways leptin also activates the sympathetic preganglionic neurons in the thoracic spinal cord. Recent studies in mice with genetic deletions of the three subtypes of adrenergic α-receptor indicate that a regulated increase in energy expenditure mediated by sympathetic nerves has in fact the capacity to affect body weight and fat stores, at least in rodents. The 'beta-less' mice were hypometabolic and slightly obese on a normal chow diet and developed severe obesity in the absence of hyperphagia when fed a high fat diet [39]. This shows that 'beta-less' mice are unable to increase energy expenditure in response to a calorically dense diet and that adrenergic activation-dependent energy expenditure contributes to the maintenance of body weight. It is unclear whether increased energy expenditure in wild-type mice is limited to brown adipose tissue or includes other sites such as muscle.

The latest concept [40] of the control of energy homeostasis by the hypothalamic neuropeptides mentioned above is that, in the basal state, catabolic neuropeptide systems are moderately activated by physiologic concentrations of leptin and insulin (see below), and that this activation is essential to prevent excessive weight gain. In contrast, anabolic pathways are inhibited by these same basal concentrations of insulin and leptin [40]. The response to weight loss includes both activation of anabolic and inhibition of catabolic pathways (fig. 2) and is, thus, more effective than the response to weight gain (stimulation of already-activated catabolic pathways and inhibition of already suppressed anabolic pathways) [40]. This concept might explain the comparatively weak effect of exogenous leptin on food intake in normal weight individuals.

For several years attention focused primarily on the neuropeptide mediators of leptin's effects, but recent findings suggest an additional mediator role of monoamines, in particular serotonin (5-HT), in this context. Serotonergic activation affects hypothalamic neuropeptide systems mediating the effects of leptin. A combination of functional neuroanatomy, feeding, and electrophysiology studies in rodents revealed that the feeding suppressive effects of d-fenfluramine requires activation of CNS melanocortin pathways. More specifically, it was shown that anorectic 5-HT drugs activate POMC neurons in the ARC through 5-HT_{2C} receptors. Furthermore, the 5-HT drug-induced hypophagia was attenuated by pharmacologic or genetic blockade of downstream melanocortin 3 and 4 receptors [41, 42]. Consistent with a role of 5-HT and the 5-HT_{2C} receptor in the feeding-inhibitory effect of leptin, we recently found that administration of a 5-HT_{2C} receptor antagonist suppressed the effect of ICV leptin in the rat [43].

Concerning the site of leptin action in the central nervous system, the original idea was that leptin would mainly, if not exclusively, act through the ARC, where receptor density is high on neurons that express the neuropeptides acting as downstream mediators of leptin. While the Arc is still considered a major site of leptin action, recent evidence indicates that also the caudal brain stem (CBS) plays an important role in the effect of leptin [44]. Thus, in situ hybridization and immunocytochemical analysis with an antibody specific to the long form of the leptin receptor revealed that this receptor is present in several rat CBS nuclei involved in the control of food intake. The CBS leptin receptors appear to be functionally relevant because in another experiment of the same study [44] fourth ICV injections of leptin reduced food intake and body weight, with both effects being indistinguishable from the effects of leptin infused into the lateral ventricle. Moreover, a ventricle-subthreshold dose of leptin microinjected unilaterally into the dorsal vagal complex suppressed food intake. Together, these results indicate that the CBS contains neurons that are direct targets for the action of leptin in the control of energy homeostasis [44].

Other Lipostatic Signals

Leptin is certainly not the only lipostatic signal. Several other hormones, such as insulin [45] and, perhaps, amylin [46] as well as some cytokines [47, 48] might have a similar function.

Amylin is a 37-amino acid peptide hormone that is co-secreted with insulin by pancreatic beta-cells in response to eating. Amylin potently reduces food intake, body weight, and adiposity when delivered into the cerebral ventricle of

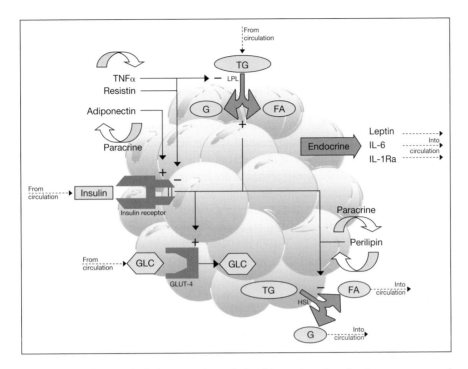

Fig. 3. Diagram depicting some interrelationships and modes of action among several adipose tissue-derived substances implicated in the control of insulin sensitivity and adiposity. FA = Fatty acids; G = glycerol; GLC = glucose; GLUT-4 = glucose transporter-4; HSL = hormone-sensitive lipase; IL-1Ra = interleukin-1 receptor antagonist; IL-6 = interleukin-6; LPL = lipoprotein lipase; TG = triglycerides; TNFα = tumor necrosis factor-α. See text for further details.

rats [46]. More importantly, ICV infusion of the specific amylin antagonist AC187 not only blocked the feeding-suppressive effect of exogenous amylin administered into the third ventricle, but chronic ICV infusion of AC187 over 14 days via implantable osmotic pumps also increased food intake throughout the test and increased body fat by about 30% [46]. In addition, adipose tissue-derived cytokines such as interleukin-6 (IL-6) and interleukin-1 receptor antagonist (IL-1Ra) may have a lipostatic function (fig. 3). IL-6 is expressed in adipose tissue in relation to adiposity. Genetically IL-6-deficient mice develop late-onset obesity that can be prevented by low-dose infusion of IL-6 into the brain [48]. Yet, it is currently unclear to what extent adipose tissue-derived IL-6 exerts an inhibitory effect on body fat. Also, it is unclear what exactly triggers cytokine production within adipose tissue. Interestingly, adipose tissue is quantitatively the most important source of the anti-inflammatory cytokine IL-1Ra

[47], and serum levels of IL-1Ra are markedly increased in obesity [49]. The obesity-related increase in IL-1Ra might contribute to central leptin resistance in obese patients similar to the inhibition of central nervous system leptin signaling by IL-1Ra in rodents [50].

Insulin has been implicated in the control of body weight for 30 years [45, 51], and it is now clear that insulin in many respects resembles leptin (fig. 1). Plasma and cerebrospinal insulin levels are proportional to adiposity, central administration of insulin reduces food intake and body weight [45, 51], and mice with a genetic deletion of neuronal insulin receptors are hyperphagic and obese [52]. Although these disturbances are less pronounced than when the leptin receptor is missing, these findings indicate that insulin receptor signaling in the CNS also plays an important role in the control of body weight and fuel metabolism. The effect of insulin on energy homeostasis could be reproduced by ICV administration of an insulin mimetic, which dose-dependently reduced food intake and body weight in rats and altered the expression of many of the same hypothalamic genes affected by leptin. Antagonism of MC-3 and MC-4 receptors reduced the effect of insulin similarly to its effect on leptin [53]. Oral administration of an insulin mimetic in a mouse model of high-fat diet-induced obesity reduced body weight gain, adiposity and insulin resistance [54]. Most evidence suggests that insulin, similar to leptin, is taken up into the brain and reaches its target neurons primarily by a receptor-mediated transport process [55]. Furthermore, insulin acts through the same hypothalamic neuropeptide systems as leptin [53], including the melanocortin system [53]. The long-term effects of insulin and leptin on food intake and body weight after ICV administration appear to be additive [56].

Finally, the recently discovered hormone ghrelin might act as a peripheral anabolic signal in the control of body weight. Ghrelin is primarily produced by endocrine cells in the stomach and is mainly known as a signal for hunger and meal initiation [57, 58]. Yet, basal plasma ghrelin levels are also increased by weight loss and decreased in obese humans [59, 60], consistent with a role of ghrelin in the lipostatic control of body weight. Ghrelin appears to act in the hypothalamus (ARC and PVN) to stimulate eating [57, 61], but it is currently unclear whether this is an endocrine effect of ghrelin produced in the stomach or a local effect of ghrelin released by neurons.

Intracellular Signaling Pathways of Leptin and Insulin

Two specific leptin-activated intracellular signals (phosphatidylinositol 3-kinase (PI3K)) [62, 63] and signal transducer and activator of transcription-3 (STAT3) [64, 65] have been identified. Interestingly, the activation of the

STAT3 pathway proved to be crucial for the control of eating but dispensable for the control of reproductive and growth axes [65]. The long form of the leptin receptor mediates activation of the transcription factor STAT3 during leptin action [66–68]. Thus, mice with a specific genetic disruption of the STAT3 signaling pathway (s/s mice) are still hyperphagic and obese, but fertile, long and less hyperglycemic than db/db mice, which are infertile, short and diabetic.

Furthermore, hypothalamic expression of NPY is elevated in db/db but not in s/s mice, whereas the hypothalamic melanocortin system is suppressed in both db/db and s/s mice. Leptin-induced STAT3 signaling thus mediates the effects of leptin on melanocortin production and body energy homeostasis, whereas distinct postreceptor signals appear to regulate NPY and the control of fertility, growth and glucose homeostasis.

As might be predicted from the above, the overlap of leptin and insulin actions on hypothalamic neurons extends to the intracellular signaling pathways [63]. Leptin and insulin signaling converges upon the insulin-receptor-substrate (IRS) PI3K pathway [62, 63, 69]. The involvement of the PI3K pathway in the feeding-suppressive effect of insulin was shown by the demonstration that ICV infusion of either of two PI3K inhibitors at doses that had no independent feeding effects prevented insulin from decreasing feeding [69]. Together with the fact that PI-3,4,5-triphosphate, the main product of PI3K activity, occurs preferentially in ARC cells that contain IRS-2, these findings support the hypothesis that the PI3K pathway is also a mediator of insulin action in the ARC and provide a plausible mechanism for neuronal cross-talk between insulin and leptin signaling.

Resistance to Leptin and Insulin

Resistance to leptin may be a major contributor to the development of obesity in humans and many rodent models [70]. Two general molecular mechanisms for leptin resistance have been identified [71]. The first may involve a defect in leptin transport across the blood brain barrier (BBB) [70, 71]. The greater potency of ICV (as opposed to peripheral) leptin to reduce food intake in mice [15] argues for a transport defect involved in resistance. The short isoforms of the leptin receptor lacking the sequences required for STAT activation are supposed to contribute to leptin transport into the CNS [72]. The impaired transport of leptin across the BBB in mice is not due to an inherently inadequate V_{max} of leptin transport; rather, the impaired leptin transport appears to develop together with obesity and appears to be reversible even with a modest weight reduction [73]. It is unresolved, however, whether leptin's actions in various regions of the hypothalamus or extra-hypothalamic brain requires transport across the BBB. If some important leptin target neurons reside outside the BBB, a defective leptin transport mechanism should not be important.

Reduced intracellular signaling may also contribute to leptin – and insulin – resistance [74]. As leptin resistance in hypothalamic neurons may occur despite an intact JAK2-STAT3 signaling pathway, a defective regulation of the PI3K pathway may as well be involved in central leptin resistance seen in obesity [74]. As mentioned above, the long isoform of the leptin receptor activates JAK/STAT signaling [66–68]. In normal mice exposed to high fat diets that promote obesity, the ability of leptin to activate STAT3 in hypothalamus is diminished [75], suggesting that impaired post-receptor signaling mechanisms contribute to leptin resistance. Also, some results indicate that SOCS3, an endogenous antagonist of leptin signaling, is rapidly induced in key hypothalamic areas by leptin [76] and contributes to leptin resistance in models of obesity.

Further Adipose Tissue-Derived Substances and Insulin Resistance

In addition to the long lipostatic feedback loop described above that controls body weight through centrally mediated modulations of energy intake and expenditure, emerging evidence suggests the existence of a local, short feedback loop that limits the size of adipocytes. Several adipose tissue-derived substances may be involved in this regulation (fig. 3).

Among the first substances to be implicated in the maintenance of body weight and metabolic efficiency were lipoprotein lipase (LPL) and tumor necrosis factor-α (TNFα). Human fat cells rely on LPL-mediated plasma triglyceride hydrolysis to store fat, and adipose tissue LPL is elevated in obesity. Muscle and adipose tissue LPL are regulated inversely, and increased adipose tissue/muscle LPL ratio partitions dietary lipid into adipose tissue. Individual differences in this ratio may explain some of the variability in weight gain when humans are exposed to excess calories [77]. Adipose tissue TNFα expression is increased in obese subjects, and TNFα may limit an increase in adipocyte size by inhibiting LPL and increasing insulin resistance [77]. A p55 TNFα receptor-mediated phosphorylation of serine residues on the insulin receptor substrate-1 appears to be an important mechanism for the effect of TNFα on insulin resistance [78, 79].

A more recently identified adipocyte-derived protein implicated in control of body weight is adiponectin. Circulating adiponectin is reduced in obesity, and this reduction is related to insulin resistance [80]. In turn, replacement of deficient adiponectin has several beneficial effects and increases insulin sensitivity [81, 82].

Adiponectin appears to act in part via a short-loop mechanism by activating the enzyme AMP kinase in adipocytes [83]. Resistin, another protein secreted by adipocytes, has also been implicated in obesity and insulin resistance [84]. Recombinant resistin has been shown to induce hepatic insulin resistance, but its exact cellular mechanism of action remains unknown [85].

The adipocyte protein perilipin, which coats adipocyte lipid droplets, was postulated to modulate hormone sensitive lipase activity and, hence, hydrolysis of stored triglycerides (TGs) [86, 87]. Mice with a genetic deletion of perilipin have normal body weight, but are leaner than controls. They display hyper- or normophygia, have increased lipolysis, and resist high-fat diet-induced obesity [86, 87]. Moreover, genetic deletion of perilipin reverses the obesity of leptin receptor deficient db/db mice by enhancing metabolism [86]. These findings suggest a role for perilipin in controlling lipolysis and energy balance.

Insulin sensitivity of adipose tissue and, hence, body fat and body weight are also influenced by peroxisome proliferator-activated receptors (PPARs). Mice heterozygous for deletion of the PPAR-γ [88, 89] are resistant to the development of obesity and have increased insulin sensitivity. On the other hand, marked activation of PPAR-γ by antidiabetic thiazoladinedione drugs also improves insulin sensitivity. This apparent discrepancy may be due to the fact that supraphysiological activation of PPAR-γ markedly increases TG content of adipose tissue, thereby decreasing TG content of liver and muscle, leading to amelioration of insulin resistance at the expense of obesity. A moderate reduction of PPAR-γ activity by heterozygous PPAR-γ deficiency decreases TG content of adipose tissue, skeletal muscle, and liver, thereby ameliorating high-fat diet-induced obesity and insulin resistance. Thus, although by different mechanisms, both heterozygous PPAR-γ deficiency and PPAR-γ agonists improve insulin resistance [90].

Many of the factors mentioned above act on body fat by influencing insulin sensitivity of adipocytes. Insulin signaling in adipocytes is necessary for the control of adipocyte size and, hence, body weight [91]. Insulin sensitivity and metabolism in adipocytes appear to be under the control of the winged helix/forkhead transcription factor gene FOXC2 and its counterpart, the FOXO1 gene, encoding the forkhead box transcription factor O1 [92, 93]. Transgenic overexpression of FOXC2 in adipocytes leads to a lean and insulin-sensitive phenotype. Increased FOXC2 levels, induced by high fat diet, seem to counteract most of the symptoms associated with obesity, including hypertriglyceridemia and diet-induced insulin resistance. In turn, genetic deficiency of the FOXO1 gene also restores insulin sensitivity by increasing adipocyte expression of insulin-sensitizing genes. These data indicate that FOXC2 and FOXO1 are positive and negative regulators of insulin sensitivity in adipocytes.

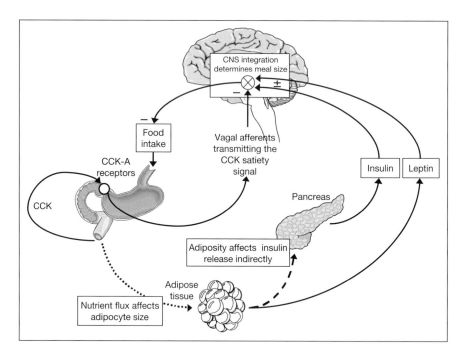

Fig. 4. Leptin and insulin act in the central nervous system (CNS) to enhance signals for meal termination produced in the gastrointestinal tract during ingestion, such as cholecystokinin (CCK). See text for further details.

From Long-Term Energy Balance to Single Meals

The meal to meal control of food intake is covered in another chapter of this book [see chapter by Gutzwiller and Beglinger, this vol., pp 1–20]. For the purpose of this chapter it therefore suffices to say that the long-term control of body weight and the short-term control of the onset and the termination of meals are closely linked. Any long-term signal which controls body weight in part by modulating food intake must ultimately modulate the frequency and/or the size of single meals. Leptin has been shown to reduce food intake by primarily affecting meal size, i.e. by enhancing the mechanisms of meal termination [94]. These findings complement what is known about pathologies of the endogenous leptin or leptin signaling system. That is, the hyperphagia of both *ob/ob* obese mice and the *fa/fa* obese rat are due to dramatic increases in meal size, with meal frequency unaffected of even reduced [95, 96]. Leptin has been shown to enhance the satiating effect of cholecystokinin (CCK) [97, 98] (fig. 4). CCK is released from the small intestine during a meal, and it reduces meal size through CCK-A receptor-mediated activation of vagal afferents which terminate in the nucleus of the solitary tract. Leptin may enhance the CCK-derived signal through descending projections from the hypothalamic PVN to these NTS neurons. In line with this concept, intraperitoneal CCK and ICV leptin administration jointly induce c-Fos expression in the PVN and the caudal brainstem, in particular in the medial nucleus of the solitary tract [99]. Interestingly, although ICV insulin also enhances the satiating potency of peripheral CCK [100], the effects of chronic insulin and leptin administration on meal patterns are slightly different. Continuous ICV infusion of 2 mU insulin/day reduced daily food intake and nocturnal meal size by amounts similar to those described for leptin, but, in contrast to the effects of chronic leptin, insulin also reduced nocturnal meal frequency [101]. Thus, it remains unclear whether the feeding effects of chronic insulin and leptin are mediated by the same mechanisms. Like the hypophagia in response to leptin and insulin, the compensatory hypophagia in response to an experimentally induced increase in body weight is mainly due to a reduction of nocturnal meal size [102]. All these findings support the hypothesis that body fat influences feeding mainly through changes in meal size. In contrast, several metabolic manipulations affect food intake by changing meal frequency rather than meal size [see 102a].

Of Women and Men

Given the marked sex differences in the incidence of obesity [103] and in the control of eating [104], it appears strange that most of the studies addressing the control of food intake and energy balance have been performed in male individuals, with the tacit assumption that the results should also be applicable to females. Only recently have researchers begun to address some of the pertinent questions also in females – with some surprising results. As far as lipostasis and body weight control are concerned, the following results deserve attention: Given the putative function of leptin as a lipostatic signal, it is interesting to note that women have substantially higher leptin levels than men of similar age at any level of adiposity [105]. This holds even for postmenopausal women, whose plasma leptin levels may be slightly higher than those in younger women [106]. Multiple regression analysis showed that adiposity and sex explain 42 and 28% of the variance of plasma leptin, respectively. Interestingly, brains of female and male rats are differentially sensitive to the feeding-inhibitory actions of small doses of these two hormones [107]. When leptin or saline was administered into the third cerebral ventricle of age- and weight-matched male and female rats, leptin significantly reduced food intake in female and male rats over 4 h, but it reduced 24-hour intake only in female rats. In contrast, insulin, administered into the cerebral ventricles, reliably reduced food intake in male rats, but not in female rats [107]. No such sex difference was observed in the sensitivity to a melanocortin agonist, however, suggesting that the sex differences in leptin and insulin sensitivities occur upstream of the melanocortin receptors. Because insulin and leptin reflect different fat beds, which are differentially distributed in males and females, the implication is that males and females regulate adiposity-relevant parameters differently.

As leptin primarily affects meal size and enhances the potency of the gastrointestinal satiety peptide CCK (see above) it is interesting to note that: (1) food intake and meal size in estrus are reduced in female rats [108]; (2) cyclic estradiol replacement reestablishes the satiety effect of CCK and the feeding-stimulatory effect of the CCK antagonist devazepide in ovariectomized rats [109], and (3) the feeding suppressive effect of endogenous CCK is more pronounced during estrus [110].

Together, these results raise the possibility that an estradiol-induced enhancement of CCK's satiety effect is an integral part of leptin's stronger suppressive effect on food intake in female individuals compared to male individuals. This hypothesis awaits experimental verification. Of course, differences in other neuropeptides, such as the MCH system, or other neurochemical mechanisms may contribute to the sex differences in the lipostatic control of food intake and body weight as well [111, 112].

Concluding Remarks

Several lines of reasoning suggest that nature tries to optimize the amount of body fat and, hence, the body weight of individuals. This theoretical prediction is confirmed by the results of numerous studies in which experimental manipulations of body weight are readily compensated by changes in energy intake and expenditure. Our understanding of the molecular pathways and physiologic systems of these weight maintenance mechanisms has increased tremendously over the last 10 years. A new peripheral adiposity signal (leptin) has been identified and central nervous system circuitries which control food intake and energy expenditure have been characterized. Several of these pathways are potential targets for drug development and may provide avenues for the pharmacological treatment of obesity. Unfortunately, however, this gain in knowledge has so far failed to prevent the steady increase in the prevalence of obesity, with all its negative consequences for human health. Thus, the present intense and exciting efforts to find pharmacologic approaches for the treatment of obesity should also be linked to the analysis and control of environmental factors that provide the basis for the current obesity epidemic, i.e. the common lack of physical activity and the wide use of foods that tend to override physiological control systems by virtue of their high palatability and high caloric density.

References

1   Hervey GR: Regulation of energy balance. Nature 1969;222:629–631.
2   Mauer MM, Harris RBS, Bartness TJ: The regulation of total body fat: Lessons learned from lipectomy studies. Neurosci Biobehav Rev 2001;25:15–28.
3   Seeley RJ, Woods SC: Monitoring of stored and available fuel by the CNS: Implications for obesity. Nat Rev Neurosci 2003;4:901–909.
4   Keesey RE, Hirvonen MD: Body weight set-points: Determination and adjustment. J Nutr 1997;127:S1875–S1883.
5   Kennedy GC: The role of depot fat in the hypothalamic control of food intake in the rat. Proc R Soc Lond [B] 1953;140:578–596.
6   Coleman DL, Hummel KP: Effects of parabiosis of normal with genetically diabetic mice. Am J Physiol 1969;217:1298–1302.
7   Coleman DL: Effects of parabiosis of obese with diabetes and normal mice. Diabetologia 1973; 9: 294–298.
8   Zhang YY, Proenca R, Maffei M, Barone M, Leopold L, Friedman JM: Positional cloning of the mouse obese gene and its human homolog. Nature 1994;372:425–432.
9   Tartaglia LA, Dembski M, Weng X, Deng NH, Culpepper J, Devos R, Richards GJ, Campfield LA, Clark FT, Deeds J, Muir C, Sanker S, Moriarty A, Moore KJ, Smutko JS, Mays GG, Woolf EA, Monroe CA, Tepper RI: Identification and expression cloning of a leptin receptor, OB-R. Cell 1995;83:1263–1271.
10 Ahima RS, Flier JS: Leptin. Ann Rev Physiol 2000;62:413–437.
11 Maffei M, Halaas J, Ravussin E, Pratley RE, Lee GH, Zhang Y, Fei H, Kim S, Lallone R, Ranganathan S, Kern PA, Friedman JM: Leptin levels in human and rodent – Measurement of plasma leptin and Ob RNA in obese and weight-reduced subjects. Nat Med 1995;1:1155–1161.
12 Considine RV, Considine EL, Williams CJ, Hyde TM, Caro JF: The hypothalamic leptin receptor in humans: Identification of incidental sequence polymorphisms and absence of the db/db mouse and fa/fa rat mutations. Diabetes 1996;45:992–994.
13 Devos R, Richards JG, Campfield LA, Tartaglia LA, Guisez Y, VanderHeyden J, Travernier J, Plaetinck G, Burn P: OB protein binds specifically to the choroid plexus of mice and rats. Proc Natl Acad Sci USA 1996;93:5668–5673.
14 Malik KF, Young WS: Localization of binding sites in the central nervous system for leptin (OB protein) in normal, obese (ob/ob), and diabetic (db/db) C57BL/6J mice. Endocrinology 1996;137:1497–1500.
15 Campfield LA, Smith FJ, Guisez Y, Devos R, Burn P: Recombinant mouse Ob protein – Evidence for a peripheral signal linking adiposity and central neural networks. Science 1995; 269:546–549.
16 Halaas JL, Gajiwala KS, Maffei M, Cohen SL, Chait BT, Rabinowitz D, Lallone RL, Burley SK, Friedman JM: Weight-reducing effects of the plasma-protein encoded by the obese gene. Science 1995;269:543–546.
17 Pelleymounter MA, Cullen MJ, Baker MB, Hecht R, Winters D, Boone T, Collins F: Effects of the obese gene-product on body-weight regulation in ob/ob mice. Science 1995;269:540–543.
18 Geary N: Endocrine controls of eating: CCK, leptin, and ghrelin. Physiol Behav 2004;82:719–733.
19 Kolaczynski JW, Considine RV, Ohannesian J, Marco C, Opentanova I, Nyce MR, Myint M, Caro JF: Responses of leptin to short-term fasting and refeeding in humans – A link with ketogenesis but not ketones themselves. Diabetes 1996;45:1511–1515.

20   Lin X, Chavez MR, Bruch RC, Kilroy GE, Simmons LA, Lin L, Braymer HD, Bray GA, York DA: The effects of a high fat diet on leptin mRNA, serum leptin and the response to leptin are not altered in a rat strain susceptible to high fat diet-induced obesity. J Nutr 1998;128:1606–1613.

21   Farooqi IS, Jebb SA, Langmack G, Lawrence E, Cheetham CH, Prentice AM, Hughes IA, McCamish MA, O'Rahilly S: Effects of recombinant leptin therapy in a child with congenital leptin deficiency. N Engl J Med 1999;341:879–884.

22   Krude H, Biebermann H, Luck W, Horn R, Brabant G, Gruters A: Severe early-onset obesity, adrenal insufficiency and red hair pigmentation caused by POMC mutations in humans. Nat Genet 1998;19:155–157.

23   Bruneau G, Vaisse C, Caraty A, Monget P: Leptin: A key for reproduction. Med Sci 1999; 15:191–196.

24   Ahima RS, Dushay J, Flier SN, Prabakaran D, Flier JS: Leptin accelerates the onset of puberty in normal female mice. J Clin Invest 1997;99:391–395.

25   Gabay C, Dreyer M, Pellegrinelli N, Chicheportiche R, Meier CA: Leptin directly induces the secretion of interleukin 1 receptor antagonist in human monocytes. J Clin Endocrinol Metab 2001;86:783–791.

26   Cohen P, Miyazaki M, Socci ND, Hagge-Greenberg A, Liedtke W, Soukas AA, Sharma R, Hudgins LC, Ntambi JM, Friedman JM: Role for stearoyl-CoA desaturase-1 in leptin-mediated weight loss. Science 2002;297:240–243.

27   Schneider JE, Zhou D, Blum RM: Leptin and metabolic control of reproduction. Horm Behav 2000;37:306–326.

28   Unger RH: Leptin physiology: A second look. Regul Peptid 2000;92:87–95.

29   Elias CF, Lee CE, Kelly JF, Ahima RS, Kuhar M, Saper CB, Elmquist JK: Characterization of CART neurons in the rat and human hypothalamus. J Comp Neurol 2001;432:1–19.

30   Elmquist JK, Marcus JN: Rethinking the central causes of diabetes. Nat Med 2003;9:645–647.

31   Morton GJ, Schwartz MW: The NPY/AgRP neuron and energy homeostasis. Int J Obes 2001; 25:S56–S62.

32   Cohen P, Zhao C, Cai XL, Montez JM, Rohani SC, Feinstein P, Mombaerts P, Friedman JM: Selective deletion of leptin receptor in neurons leads to obesity. J Clin Invest 2001;108: 1113–1121.

33   Schwartz MW, Woods SC, Porte D, Seeley RJ, Baskin DG: Central nervous system control of food intake. Nature 2000;404:661–671.

34   Elmquist JK: Hypothalamic pathways underlying the endocrine, autonomic, and behavioral effects of leptin. Int J Obes 2001;25:S78–S82.

35   Kristensen P, Judge ME, Thim L, Ribel U, Christjansen KN, Wulff BS, Clausen JT, Jensen PB, Madsen OD, Vrang N, Larsen PJ, Hastrup S: Hypothalamic CART is a new anorectic peptide regulated by leptin. Nature 1998;393:72–76.

36   Zheng HY, Corkern MM, Crousillac SM, Patterson LM, Phifer CB, Berthoud HR: Neurochemical phenotype of hypothalamic neurons showing Fos expression 23 h after intracranial AgRP. Am J Physiol 2002;282:R1773–R1781.

37   Olszewski PK, Wirth MM, Grace MK, Levine AS, Giraudo SQ: Evidence of interactions between melanocortin and opioid systems in regulation of feeding. Neuroreport 2001;12:1727–1730.

38   Boutin JA, Suply T, Audinot V, Rodriguez M, Beauverger P, Nicolas JP, Galizzi JP, Fauchere JL: Melanin-concentrating hormone and its receptors: State of the art. Can J Physiol Pharmacol 2002;80:388–395.

39   Bachman ES, Dhillon H, Zhang CY, Cinti S, Bianco AC, Kobilka BK, Lowell BB: Beta AR signaling required for diet-induced thermogenesis and obesity resistance. Science 2002;297:843–845.

40   Schwartz MW, Woods SC, Seeley RJ, Barsh GS, Baskin DG, Leibel RL: Is the energy homeostasis system inherently biased toward weight gain? Diabetes 2003;52:232–238.

41   Heisler LK, Cowley MA, Tecott LH, Fan W, Low MJ, Smart JL, Rubinstein M, Tatro JB, Marcus JN, Holstege H, Lee CE, Cone RD, Elmquist JK: Activation of central melanocortin pathways by fenfluramine. Science 2002;297:609–611.

42   Heisler LK, Cowley MA, Kishi T, Tecott LH, Fan W, Low MJ, Smart JL, Rubinstein M, Tatro JB, Zigman JM, Cone RD, Elmquist JK: Central serotonin and melanocortin pathways regulating energy homeostasis. Melanocortin System. Ann NY Acad Sci 2003;994:169–174.

43   von Meyenburg C, Langhans W, Hrupka BJ: Evidence for a role of the 5-HT2C receptor in central lipopolysaccharide-, interleukin-1 beta-, and leptin-induced anorexia. Pharmacol Biochem Behav 2003;74:1025–1031.

44   Grill HJ, Schwartz MW, Kaplan JM, Foxhall JS, Breininger J, Baskin DG: Evidence that the caudal brainstem is a target for the inhibitory effect of leptin on food intake. Endocrinology 2002; 143:239–246.

45   Woods SC, Seeley RJ: Insulin as an adiposity signal. Int J Obes 2001;25:S35–S38.

46   Rushing PA, Hagan MM, Seeley RJ, Lutz TA, D'Alessio DA, Air EL, Woods SC: Inhibition of central amylin signaling increases food intake and body adiposity in rats. Endocrinology 2001; 142:5035–5038.

47   Juge-Aubry CE, Somm E, Giusti V, Pernin A, Chicheportiche R, Verdumo C, Rohner-Jeanrenaud F, Burger D, Dayer JM, Meier CA: Adipose tissue is a major source of interleukin-1 receptor antagonist: Upregulation in obesity and inflammation. Diabetes 2003;52:1104–1110.

48   Wallenius V, Wallenius K, Ahren B, Rudling M, Carlsten H, Dickson SL, Ohlsson C, Jansson JO: Interleukin-6-deficient mice develop mature-onset obesity. Nat Med 2002;8:75–79.

49   Meier CA, Bobbioni E, Gabay C, Assimacopoulos-Jeannet F, Golay A, Dayer JM: IL-1 receptor antagonist serum levels are increased in human obesity: A possible link to the resistance to leptin? J Clin Endocrinol Metab 2002;87:1184–1188.

50   Luheshi GN, Gardner JD, Rushforth DA, Loudon AS, Rothwell NJ: Leptin actions on food intake and body temperature are mediated by IL-1. Proc Natl Acad Sci USA 1999;96:7047–7052.

51   Woods SC, Decke E, Vasselli JR: Metabolic hormones and regulation of body weight. Psychol Rev 1974;81:26–43.

52   Bruning JC, Gautam D, Burks DJ, Gillette J, Schubert M, Orban PC, Klein R, Krone W, Muller-Wieland D, Kahn CR: Role of brain insulin receptor in control of body weight and reproduction. Science 2000;289:2122–2125.

53   Benoit SC, Air EL, Coolen LM, Strauss R, Jackman A, Clegg DJ, Seeley RJ, Woods SC: The catabolic action of insulin in the brain is mediated by melanocortins. J Neurosci 2002;22:9048–9052.

54   Air EL, Strowski MZ, Benoit SC, Conarello SL, Salituro GM, Guan XM, Liu K, Woods SC, Zhang BB: Small molecule insulin mimetics reduce food intake and body weight and prevent development of obesity. Nat Med 2002;8:179–183.

55   Woods SC, Seeley RJ, Baskin DG, Schwartz MW: Insulin and the blood-brain barrier. Curr Pharm Design 2003;9:795–800.

56   Air EL, Benoit SC, Clegg DJ, Seeley RJ, Woods SC: Insulin and leptin combine additively to reduce food intake and body weight in rats. Endocrinology 2002;143:2449–2452.

57   Wren AM, Small CJ, Abbott CR, Dhillo WS, Seal LJ, Cohen MA, Batterham RL, Taheri S, Stanley SA, Ghatei MA, Bloom SR: Ghrelin causes hyperphagia and obesity in rats. Diabetes 2001;50:2540–2547.

58   Wren AM, Seal LJ, Cohen MA, Brynes AE, Frost GS, Murphy KG, Dhillo WS, Ghatei MA, Bloom SR: Ghrelin enhances appetite and increases food intake in humans. J Clin Endocrinol Metab 2001;86:5992–5995.

59   Cummings DE, Weigle DS, Frayo RS, Breen PA, Ma MK, Dellinger EP, Purnell JQ: Plasma ghrelin levels after diet-induced weight loss or gastric bypass surgery. N Engl J Med 2002;346:1623–1630.

60   Tschop M, Weyer C, Tataranni PA, Devanarayan V, Ravussin E, Heiman ML: Circulating ghrelin levels are decreased in human obesity. Diabetes 2001;50:707–709.

61   Bagnasco M, Tulipano G, Melis MR, Argiolas A, Cocchi D, Muller EE: Endogenous ghrelin is an orexigenic peptide acting in the arcuate nucleus in response to fasting. Regul Pept 2003;111:161–167.

62   Niswender KD, Morton GJ, Stearns WH, Rhodes CJ, Myers MG, Schwartz MW: Intracellular signalling – Key enzyme in leptin-induced anorexia. Nature 2001;413:794–795.

63   Niswender KD, Schwartz MW: Insulin and leptin revisited: Adiposity signals with overlapping physiological and intracellular signaling capabilities. Front Neuroendocrinol 2003;24:1–10.

64   Bates SH, Myers MG: The role of leptin receptor signaling in feeding and neuroendocrine function. Trends Endocrinol Metab 2003;14:447–452.

65   Bates SH, Stearns WH, Dundon TA, Schubert M, Tso AWK, Wang YP, Banks AS, Lavery HJ, Haq AK, Maratos-Flier E, Neel BG, Schwartz MW, Myers MG: STAT3 signalling is required for leptin regulation of energy balance but not reproduction. Nature 2003;421:856–859.

66 Baumann H, Morella KK, White DW, Dembski M, Bailon PS, Kim HK, Lai CF, Tartaglia LA: The full-length leptin receptor has signaling capabilities of interleukin 6-type cytokine receptors. Proc Natl Acad Sci USA 1996;93:8374–8378.

67 Vaisse C, Halaas JL, Horvath CM, Darnell JE, Stoffel M, Friedman JM: Leptin activation of Stat3 in the hypothalamus of wildtype and ob/ob mice but not db/db mice. Nat Genet 1996;14:95–97.

68 White DW, Kuropatwinski KK, Devos R, Baumann H, Tartaglia LA: Leptin receptor (OBR) signaling – Cytoplasmic domain mutational analysis and evidence for receptor homooligomerization. J Biol Chem 1997;272:4065–4071.

69 Niswender KD, Morrison CD, Clegg DJ, Olson R, Baskin DG, Myers MG, Seeley RJ, Schwartz MW: Insulin activation of phosphatidylinositol 3-kinase in the hypothalamic arcuate nucleus – A key mediator of insulin-induced anorexia. Diabetes 2003;52:227–231.

70 Banks WA: Leptin transport across the blood-brain barrier: Implications for the cause and treatment of obesity. Curr Pharm Design 2001;7:125–133.

71 Flier JS: Obesity wars: Molecular progress confronts an expanding epidemic. Cell 2004;116: 337–350.

72 Hileman SM, Pierroz DD, Masuzaki H, Bjorbaek C, El Haschimi K, Banks WA, Flier JS: Characterization of short isoforms of the leptin receptor in rat cerebral microvessels and of brain uptake of leptin in mouse models of obesity. Endocrinology 2002;143:775–783.

73 Banks WA, Farrell CL: Impaired transport of leptin across the blood-brain barrier in obesity is acquired and reversible. Am J Physiol 2003;285:E10–E15.

74 Sahu A: Leptin signaling in the hypothalamus: Emphasis on energy homeostasis and leptin resistance. Front Neuroendocrinol 2003;24:225–253.

75 El Haschimi K, Pierroz DD, Hileman SM, Bjorbaek C, Flier JS: Two defects contribute to hypothalamic leptin resistance in mice with diet-induced obesity. J Clin Invest 2000;105: 1827–1832.

76 Bjorbaek C, El Haschimi K, Frantz JD, Flier JS: The role of SOCS-3 in leptin signaling and leptin resistance. J Biol Chem 1999;274:30059–30065.

77 Kern PA: Potential role of TNF alpha and lipoprotein lipase as candidate genes for obesity. J Nutr 1997;127:S1917–S1922.

78 Hotamisligil GS: Mechanisms of TNF-alpha-induced insulin resistance. Exp Clin Endocrinol Diab 1999;107:119–125.

79 Uysal KT, Wiesbrock SM, Hotamisligil GS: Functional analysis of tumor necrosis factor (TNF) receptors in TNF-alpha-mediated insulin resistance in genetic obesity. Endocrinology 1998;139:4832–4838.

80 Weyer C, Funahashi T, Tanaka S, Hotta K, Matsuzawa Y, Pratley RE, Tataranni PA: Hypo-adiponectinemia in obesity and type 2 diabetes: Close association with insulin resistance and hyperinsulinemia. J Clin Endocrinol Metab 2001;86:1930–1935.

81 Berg AH, Combs TP, Du X, Brownlee M, Scherer PE: The adipocyte-secreted protein Acrp30 enhances hepatic insulin action. Nat Med 2001;7:947–953.

82 Shklyaev S, Aslanidi G, Tennant M, Prima V, Kohlbrenner E, Kroutov V, Campbell-Thompson M, Crawford J, Shek EW, Scarpace PJ, Zolotukhin S: Sustained peripheral expression of transgene adiponectin offsets the development of diet-induced obesity in rats. Proc Natl Acad Sci USA 2003;100:14217–14222.

83 Yamauchi T, Kamon J, Minokoshi Y, Ito Y, Waki H, Uchida S, Yamashita S, Noda M, Kita S, Ueki K, Eto K, Akanuma Y, Froguel P, Foufelle F, Ferre P, Carling D, Kimura S, Nagai R, Kahn BB, Kadowaki T: Adiponectin stimulates glucose utilization and fatty-acid oxidation by activating AMP-activated protein kinase. Nat Med 2002;8:1288–1295.

84 Steppan CM, Bailey ST, Bhat S, Brown EJ, Banerjee RR, Wright CM, Patel HR, Ahima RS, Lazar MA: The hormone resistin links obesity to diabetes. Nature 2001;409:307–312.

85 Way JM, Gorgun CZ, Tong Q, Uysal KT, Brown KK, Harrington WW, Oliver WR Jr., Willson TM, Kliewer SA, Hotamisligil GS: Adipose tissue resistin expression is severely suppressed in obesity and stimulated by peroxisome proliferator-activated receptor gamma agonists. J Biol Chem 2001;276:25651–25653.

86 Martinez-Botas J, Anderson JB, Tessier D, Lapillonne A, Chang BH, Quast MJ, Gorenstein D, Chen KH, Chan L: Absence of perilipin results in leanness and reverses obesity in Lepr(db/db) mice. Nat Genet 2000;26:474–479.

87 Tansey JT, Sztalryd C, Gruia-Gray J, Roush DL, Zee JV, Gavrilova O, Reitman ML, Deng CX, Li C, Kimmel AR, Londos C: Perilipin ablation results in a lean mouse with aberrant adipocyte lipolysis, enhanced leptin production, and resistance to diet-induced obesity. Proc Natl Acad Sci USA 2001;98:6494–6499.

88 Miles PDG, Barak Y, He WM, Evans RM, Olefsky JM: Improved insulin-sensitivity in mice heterozygous for PPAR-gamma deficiency. J Clin Invest 2000;105:287–292.

89 Yamauchi T, Waki H, Kamon J, Murakami K, Motojima K, Komeda K, Miki H, Kubota N, Terauchi Y, Tsuchida A, Tsuboyama-Kasaoka N, Yamauchi N, Ide T, Hori W, Kato S, Fukayama M, Akanuma Y, Ezaki O, Itai A, Nagai R, Kimura S, Tobe K, Kagechika H, Shudo K, Kadowaki T: Inhibition of RXR and PPAR gamma ameliorates diet-induced obesity and type 2 diabetes. J Clin Invest 2001;108:1001–1013.

90 Yamauchi T, Kamon J, Waki H, Murakami K, Motojima K, Komeda K, Ide T, Kubota N, Terauchi Y, Tobe K, Miki H, Tsuchida A, Akanuma Y, Nagai R, Kimura S, Kadowaki T: Mechanisms by which both heterozygous peroxisome proliferator-activated receptor gamma (PPAR gamma) deficiency and PPAR gamma agonist improve insulin resistance. J Biol Chem 2001;276:41245–41254.

91 Bluher M, Michael MD, Peroni OD, Ueki K, Carter N, Kahn BB, Kahn CR: Adipose tissue selective insulin receptor knockout protects against obesity and obesity-related glucose intolerance. Dev Cell 2002;3:25–38.

92 Cederberg A, Gronning LM, Ahren B, Tasken K, Carlsson P, Enerback S: FOXC2 is a winged helix gene that counteracts obesity, hypertriglyceridemia, and diet-induced insulin resistance. Cell 2001;106:563–573.

93 Nakai J, Biggs WH, Kitamura T, Cavenee WK, Wright CVE, Arden KC, Accili D: Regulation of insulin action and pancreatic beta-cell function by mutated alleles of the gene encoding forkhead transcription factor Foxo1. Nat Genet 2002;32:245–253.

94 Kahler A, Eckel LA, Geary N, Campfield LA, Smith FJ, Langhans W: Chronic administration of OB protein decreases spontaneous food intake by reducing meal size in male rats. Am J Physiol 1998;275:R180–R185.

95 Alingh PA, Jong-Nagelsmit A, Keijser J, Strubbe JH: Daily rhythms of feeding in the genetically obese and lean Zucker rats. Physiol Behav 1986;38:423–426.

96 Strohmayer AJ, Smith GP: The meal pattern of genetically obese (ob/ob) mice. Appetite 1987; 8:111–123.

97 Barrachina MD, Martinez V, Wang LX, Wei JY, Tache Y: Synergistic interaction between leptin and cholecystokinin to reduce short-term food intake in lean mice. Proc Natl Acad Sci USA 1997;94:10455–10460.

98 Emond M, Schwartz GJ, Ladenheim EE, Moran TH: Central leptin modulates behavioral and neural responsivity to CCK. Am J Physiol 1999;276:R1545–R1549.

99 Blevins JE, Schwartz MW, Baskin DG: Peptide signals regulating food intake and energy homeostasis. Can J Physiol Pharmacol 2002;80:396–406.

100 Riedy CA, Chavez M, Figlewicz DP, Woods SC: Central insulin enhances sensitivity to cholecystokinin. Physiol Behav 1995;58:755–760.

101 Plata-Salamàn CR, Oomura Y, Shimizu N: Dependence of food intake on acute and chronic ventricular administration of insulin. Physiol Behav 1986;37:717–734.

102 Geary N, Grötschel H, Petry HP, Scharrer E: Meal patterns and body weight changes during insulin hyperphagia and postinsulin hypophagia. Behav Neural Biol 1981;31:435–442.

102a Langhans W: Role of the liver in the metabolic control of eating: what we know – and what we do not know. Neurosci Biobehav Rev 1996;20:145–153.

103 Flegal KM, Carroll MD, Ogden CL, Johnson CL: Prevalence and trends in obesity among US adults, 1999–2000. J Am Med Assoc 2002;288:1723–1727.

104 Geary N: Is the control of fat ingestion sexually differentiated? Physiol Behav, in press.

105 Saad MF, Damani S, Gingerich RL, RiadGabriel MG, Khan A, Boyadjian R, Jinagouda SD, ElTawil K, Rude RK, Kamdar V: Sexual dimorphism in plasma leptin concentration. J Clin Endocrinol Metab 1997;82:579–584.

106 Rosenbaum M, Nicolson M, Hirsch J, Heymsfield SB, Gallagher D, Chu F, Leibel RL: Effects of gender, body composition, and menopause on plasma concentrations of leptin. J Clin Endocrinol Metab 1996;81:3424–3427.

107 Clegg DJ, Riedy CA, Smith KAB, Benoit SC, Woods SC: Differential sensitivity to central leptin and insulin in male and female rats. Diabetes 2003;52:682–687.
108 Geary N, Asarian L: Cyclic estradiol treatment normalizes body weight and test meal size in ovariectomized rats. Physiol Behav 1999;67:141–147.
109 Asarian L, Geary N: Cyclic estradiol treatment phasically potentiates endogenous cholecystokinin's satiating action in ovariectomized rats. Peptides 1999;20:445–450.
110 Eckel LA, Geary N: Endogenous cholecystokinin's satiating action increases during estrus in female rats. Peptides 1999;20:451–456.
111 Ishii M, Fei H, Friedman JM: Targeted disruption of GPR7, the endogenous receptor for neuropeptides B and W, leads to metabolic defects and adult-onset obesity. Proc Natl Acad Sci USA 2003;100:10540–10545.
112 Mystkowski P, Schwartz MW: Gonadal steroids and energy homeostasis in the leptin era. Nutrition 2000;16:937–946.

Prof. Wolfgang Langhans
Institut für Nutztierwissenschaften
ETH-Aussenstation Schwerzenbach, Schorenstrasse 16
CH–8603 Schwerzenbach (Switzerland)
Tel. +41 1 655 7420, Fax +41 1 655 7206, E-Mail wolfgang.langhans@inw.agrl.ethz.ch

Munsch S, Beglinger C (eds): Obesity and Binge Eating Disorder.
Bibl Psychiatr. Basel, Karger, 2005, No 171, pp 41–61

Epidemiology and Symptomatology of Obesity

Johannes Georg Wechsler[a]*, Kristine Leopold*[b]*, Gert Bischoff*[a]

[a]Krankenhaus Barmherzige Brüder, München, Germany; [b]Centre Hospitalier Universitaire Vaudois, Service de Gastro-Entérologie et d'Hépatologie, Lausanne, Switzerland

Overweight and obesity are clearly defined classifications (table 1) [5, 8, 18, 27, 30]. These two conditions are dramatically increasing in countries having an abundance of high calorie food products and low tendency to exercise. According to the World Health Organization, being overweight for a longer period of time and exceeding certain threshold values leads to disease [30]. Numerous diseases arise from being overweight and obese, and these lead to infirmities, limit the quality of life and lower life expectancy [11, 19, 20]. With android fat distribution, obesity is associated with a high risk for many diseases [7b], while gynoid fat distribution, as frequently seen in women, has a clearly lower risk of associated disease [5, 8, 18, 27, 30].

Overweight and Obesity Classification

The body mass index is the most widely used measure for classifying the various degrees of being overweight, and is calculated by dividing the weight in kg by the height in m².

The World Health Organization (WHO), the National Institute of Health (NIH) and the German Obesity Society (Deutsche Adipositas-Gesellschaft – DAG) recommend using an age- and gender-independent body mass index [8, 18, 30]. The waist-to-hip ratio, another good parameter for differentiating between android or gynoid fat distribution, is also used in risk assessment. When the waist circumference is >88 cm in women or >102 cm in men, abdominal obesity is present. When the body mass index is >25, the waist circumference should always be measured [18].

Table 1. Classification of obesity based on BMI (WHO and DAG)

	BMI, kg/m^2
Normal weight	20–25
Overweight	25–30
Obesity I	30–35
Obesity II	35–40
Obesity III	>40

When bioelectric impedance analysis is used to measure the body fat mass, the results contain a non-calculable margin of error. With this technique, one actually measures electric conductivity rather than body fat. Calculating the body fat mass using magnetic resonance imaging (MRI) is very expensive and rather complex. Better results are reported with the DEXA method (dual-energy X-ray absorptiometry), and precise results are also returned by a calculation that involves determining the density using the measurement of body water (densitometry) [29].

Among children and adolescents, both age- and gender-specific changes of the BMI must be considered. For overweight and obesity determinations in this population, it is better to follow the gender-specific age percentiles for the BMI.

According to the guidelines of the German AGA study group (AGA: Arbeitsgemeinschaft Adipositas im Kindes- und Jugendalter = Working Group, Obesity in Childhood and Adolescence), there are no defined values for the health hazard posed by body fat mass for youths. In contrast to adults, the incidence of obesity-related diseases is low in children and adolescents, and there is also a lack of sufficient longitudinal studies investigating the health risk of obesity among the young. The AGA recommends using the body mass index for evaluating overweight states and obesity in childhood and adolescence, just as they do in adulthood. The percentiles presented here are to be used as reference values for German children. The determination of overweight or obesity should follow using the 90th and 97th, age- and gender-specific percentiles from these reference data (fig. 1). The Expert Committee convened by the International Obesity Task Force (IOTF) recommends using BMI percentiles for defining children or adolescents as being overweight or obese. At the age of 18 years, these BMI percentiles for overweight or obesity equal 25 and 30 kg/m^2, respectively, and thus correspond to the risk-related values for adults [1, 30].

In accordance with the established procedures for classifying biological parameters in children and adolescents, the statistical distribution of reference values is also used for the BMI, and exceeding the 90th percentile (one standard

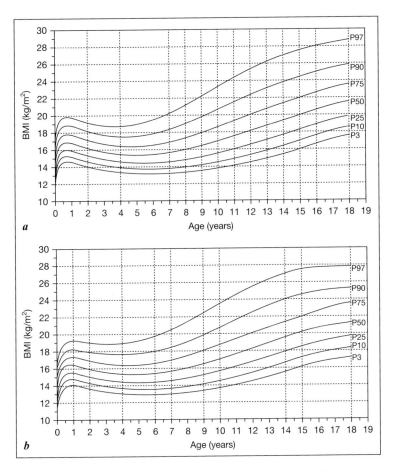

Fig. 1. Body mass index percentiles of boys (**a**) and girls (**b**) between 0 and 18 years of age [1] (90th to 97th percentile).

deviation) or the 97th percentile (two standard deviations) is described as conspicuous, respectively, very conspicuous. Following the guidelines from the European Childhood Obesity Group (ECOG), the AGA recommends using the 90th and 97th age- and gender-specific percentiles from the reference data presented above as limits for defining being overweight or obese. When the new references for German children and adolescents are used, this purely statistical threshold determination enables an almost continuous transition to the above-cited values for adults.

Epidemiology of Obesity in Children and Adolescents

When using the age- and gender-specific 90th and 97th percentiles of the normal distribution, some 10–20% of schoolchildren and adolescents in Europe and the USA are overweight or obese [1, 30] (fig. 4).

In the new German states (formerly East Germany), one sees that the frequency of obesity correlates with the social status. Among girls from a lower social status, 16.1% were obese while among those from a higher social status, this figure was 10.4%. These results are also seen in men and women. Figure 2 shows that obesity and being overweight negatively correlate with social status.

In the USA, the National Health and Nutrition Examination Survey (NHANES III) found 15.5% of 12- to 19-year-olds were overweight; 15.3% of 6- to 11-year-olds, and 10.4% of 2- to 5-year-olds. Comparative data from the years 1976 to 1980 were 10.5, 11.3 and 7.2%, respectively, indicating an approximate 50% increase in about 20 years [13, 23].

More recent data from NHANES 1999–2002 [13] show a clear disparity in the frequency of being overweight and obese among the various ethnic groups. For example, the frequency of being overweight was significantly higher in Mexican-American boys than in non-Hispanic white and black boys. In adults, this difference was not detectable. The frequency of being overweight for girls who entered the study at 6 years of age, as well as the prevalence of obesity for women of all age groups, was significantly higher for non-Hispanic blacks than for non-Hispanic whites. Even Mexican-American girls had no significantly lower prevalence of being overweight than non-Hispanic black girls (fig. 3a, b) [23]. Nevertheless, the frequency of obesity among Mexican-American women was significantly lower than in non-Hispanic black women.

In the years 1989–1998 in England, Bundred et al. [6] prospectively examined 64,000 babies in the 4th–12th week and young children between 2.9 and 4 years of age. They found a significant increase in the frequency of overweight children. In these 10 years, the frequency of overweight young children rose from 14.7 to 23.6%, and the frequency of obesity increased from 5.4% on 9.2%. Among babies, there was a trend toward weight gain.

The primary causes for being overweight and obese are the nearly unlimited access to food throughout the entire world, the drastic reduction in physical activity, as well as the fulfillment of the genetic response that the body store up fat reserves during times of abundance for 'leaner' periods later on. The easy availability of food (fast food) presents an additional significant factor. A decline in physical activity has been shown for adolescents and adults. Likewise, women are less active than men, and more black women than white women indicate a lower level of physical activity [30].

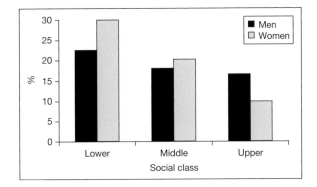

Fig. 2. Frequency of obesity among 18- to 79-year-old men and women, classified according to social status [12].

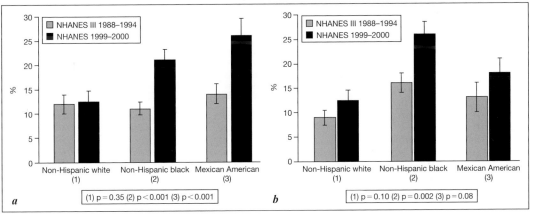

Fig. 3. *a* Overweight prevalence by race/ethnicity for adolescent boys [23]. *b* Overweight prevalence by race/ethnicity for adolescent girls [23].

Epidemiology of Obesity in Adults

In the Federal Republic of Germany, normal weight is seen in only about one-third of the male population; among women, in less than half. Accordingly, more than half the population is overweight, approximately 20% are obese [12].

When age groups are considered, in both men and women, being overweight or obese rises with increasing age (fig. 5). In former West Germany

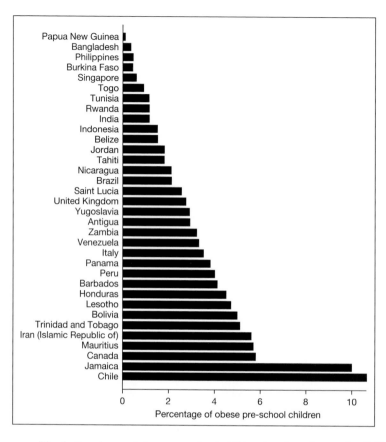

Fig. 4. Prevalence of obese pre-school children in selected countries [30].

between 1991 and 1998, the prevalence of obesity among men 25 to 69 years of age rose from 17.4 to 19.4% and from 20.6 to 21.8% in former East Germany. Among women, the frequency of obesity in former West Germany rose from 19.6 to 20.9%, while in former East Germany, it actually fell from 25.8 to 24.2%. Figure 6 shows that overweight and obesity is more frequent in former East Germany.

In Europe, obesity is found, on average, between 10 and 20% of men, and 10 and 25% of women. In England between 1980 and 1995, the frequency of obesity rose from 6 to 15% in men, and from 8 to 16% in women. The lowest increase is reported by the Netherlands where, in 1987, 6% of the men and 8% of the women were obese; in 1995, it was 8% of both men and women. There is as yet no explanation for the phenomenon that, in the Netherlands and Sweden, the frequency of obesity clearly lies lower than in other European countries [30].

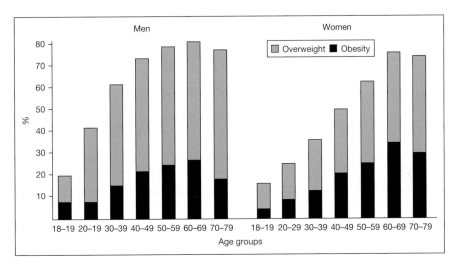

Fig. 5. Percentage of men and women in various age groups who are overweight or obese [12].

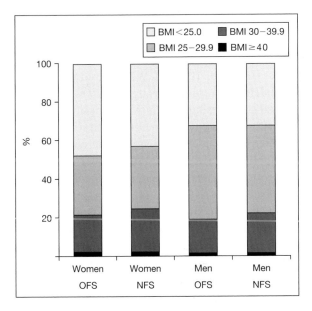

Fig. 6. Body mass index (men and women 18–79 years of age) in OFS (former West Germany) and NFS (former East Germany) [12].

Table 2. Percentage of overweight and obese in the population (WHO 1998)

USA	65
Germany	60
Russia	60–80
Italy	50
France	40
China	40

The trends noted in the Germany are seen even more blatantly in the USA where, in 1960, 30.5% of the population was overweight; today, it is more than 60% (table 2, fig. 9) [21]. Among a selection representative of the US population in the years 1960 to 2000, the National Health and Nutrition Examination Survey (NHANES I to III) showed a significant increase in the rate of overweight and obese. The percentage of those suffering from obesity, i.e. a body mass index above 30, was 13.4% in 1960, rose to 14.5% in 1973, to 15% in 1980, to 23% in 1994, and at the last investigation in the year 2000, to almost 31%. This tendency could be observed in both men and women and was even more prevalent among younger age groups. Grade III obesity (morbid obesity) with a BMI above 40 climbed significantly from 2.9 to 4.7% [10, 30]. The rising frequency in obesity leads to increasing morbidity and mortality. Thus in the USA, approximately 280,000 annual deaths are attributable to obesity [2].

An overview of the frequency of obesity can best be obtained from the WHO MONICA Study (table 2) (fig. 7, 8, 10) [30]. When worldwide prevalence rates are considered, a tendency toward increasing obesity is detectable not only in western, industrialized countries but also in Africa, despite regional food shortages. In particular, with an increase in socio-economic status and urbanization, black African women show an extreme increase in obesity; 44% of African women who live in South Africa are obese [30].

Besides the USA, Canada as well as increasing numbers of South American countries, such as Brazil, are affected by a rise in the prevalence of obesity. In Brazil between 1975 and 1989, the frequency of obesity in Brazilian men climbed from 3 to 6%, and in women from 8 to 13%. In the USA from 1960 to 1991, obesity rates in men rose from 10 to 20% and in women, from 15 to 25%. The tremendous increase of obesity in the United States can be seen in figure 9 [21, 22]. Likewise in the Caribbean countries of Barbados, Cuba, Jamaica and St. Lucia, as the GNP increases, one sees a similar increase in obesity, more so among women than men. Similar data are reported from Asia, e.g. Thailand. Even in China, there is an unmistakable tendency toward increased body weight.

Among married women in the United Arab Emirates, the frequency of obesity is about 40% and in married men, about 16% [30]. In Kuwait, the

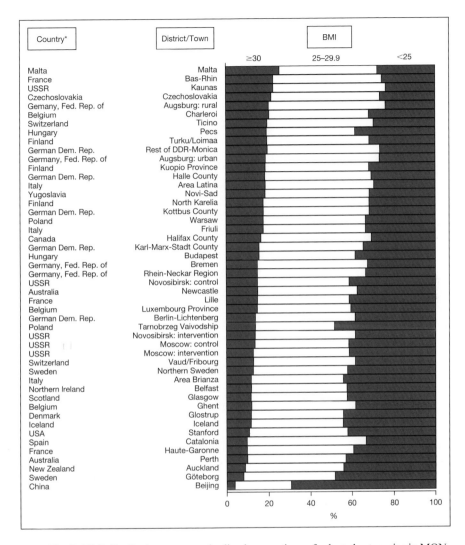

The chart columns:

Country*	District/Town	BMI ≥30	BMI 25–29.9	BMI <25
Malta	Malta			
France	Bas-Rhin			
USSR	Kaunas			
Czechoslovakia	Czechoslovakia			
Gemany, Fed. Rep. of	Augsburg: rural			
Belgium	Charleroi			
Switzerland	Ticino			
Hungary	Pecs			
Finland	Turku/Loimaa			
German Dem. Rep.	Rest of DDR-Monica			
Germany, Fed. Rep. of	Augsburg: urban			
Finland	Kuopio Province			
German Dem. Rep.	Halle County			
Italy	Area Latina			
Yugoslavia	Novi-Sad			
Finland	North Karelia			
German Dem. Rep.	Kottbus County			
Poland	Warsaw			
Italy	Friuli			
Canada	Halifax County			
German Dem. Rep.	Karl-Marx-Stadt County			
Hungary	Budapest			
Germany, Fed. Rep. of	Bremen			
Germany, Fed. Rep. of	Rhein-Neckar Region			
USSR	Novosibirsk: control			
Australia	Newcastle			
France	Lille			
Belgium	Luxembourg Province			
German Dem. Rep.	Berlin-Lichtenberg			
Poland	Tarnobrzeg Vaivodship			
USSR	Novosibirsk: intervention			
USSR	Moscow: control			
USSR	Moscow: intervention			
Switzerland	Vaud/Fribourg			
Sweden	Northern Sweden			
Italy	Area Brianza			
Northern Ireland	Belfast			
Scotland	Glasgow			
Belgium	Ghent			
Denmark	Glostrup			
Iceland	Iceland			
USA	Stanford			
Spain	Catalonia			
France	Haute-Garonne			
Australia	Perth			
New Zealand	Auckland			
Sweden	Göteborg			
China	Beijing			

Fig. 7. BMI distribution: age-standardized proportions of selected categories in MONICA populations, age group 35–64 years (men) [30].

highest numbers are recorded with a prevalence rate of 32% in men and 44% in women [30]. Two extreme examples can be reported from the western Pacific region. In 1976 Japan, 0.7% of the men and 2.8% of the women were obese; in 1993, only 1.8% of the men and 2.6% of the women. In contrast to Japan, excessively frequent cases of obesity have been reported from Samoa, particularly in urban areas. Between 1978 and 1991, the frequency of obesity in men

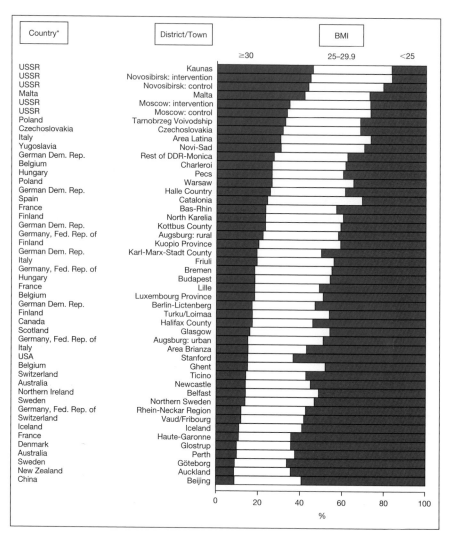

Fig. 8. BMI distribution: age-standardized proportions of selected categories in MON-ICA populations, age group 35–64 years (women) [30].

rose from 39 to 58%, and in women from 59 to 77%. The BMI distribution of various adult populations worldwide is shown in figure 10 [30].

The trend showing an increase in the overweight population can be seen throughout the world, and with it, the manifestations of being overweight and obese. Frequency rates, such as those presented in table 2 and figures 7–9, impel the WHO to speak of an epidemic of obesity and to classify obesity as a chronic disease [30].

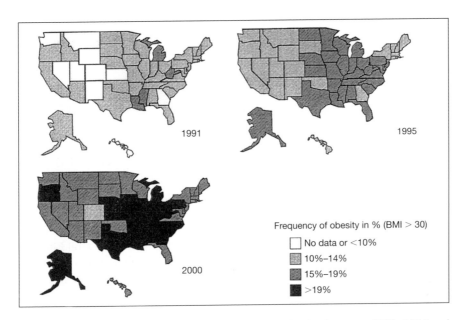

Frequency of obesity in % (BMI > 30)

- No data or <10%
- 10%–14%
- 15%–19%
- >19%

Fig. 9. Percentage of obese population in the USA in the years 1991, 1995 and 2000 [21].

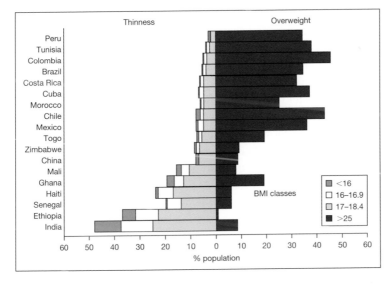

Fig. 10. BMI distribution of various adult populations worldwide (both sexes) [30].

The obese suffer not only from a heavier psychological burden, but are also discriminated against socially. As a result, a negative correlation exists between obesity and social status (fig. 2) [12].

Symptomatology of Being Overweight and Obese

Somatic and Psychological Consequences of Obesity in Adults

Being overweight and obese leads to numerous associated diseases (table 3), but even without the accompanying so-called risk factors, being overweight and obese evoke an increased risk of mortality (fig. 14, 15) [17]. However, together with associated diseases (table 3), the risk climbs exponentially. Almost unconditionally, obesity leads to the complete picture of the metabolic syndrome. As clearly defined by the World Health Organization [30], the metabolic syndrome includes hypertension, dyslipidemia or hyperlipidemia, adiposity and microalbuminuria. However, the metabolic syndrome also includes the clinical manifestations of android obesity, i.e. disturbed glucose tolerance, type II diabetes, dyslipidemia, hypertension, premature arteriosclerosis, hyperuricemia and gout; androgenism in women leads to osteoporosis and albuminuria, hypercoagulation, fibrinolysis defects, sleep apnea and fatty liver.

High blood pressure very frequently accompanies adiposity. There is a positive correlation between BMI and the frequency of hypertension. High blood pressure is an acknowledged risk factor for coronary heart disease (CHD), premature development of arteriosclerosis and stroke [18]. The PROCAM Study plainly shows that arterial hypertension is clearly more frequent among men (48%) and women (47%) having a BMI >30 than among men and women of normal weight (8%) [3].

The risk for heart attacks climbs with increasing weight. The relative risk for developing CHD among those having a BMI between 25 and 29 is twice as high as among those of normal weight. With a BMI above 29, the disease risk is three times higher. The Framingham Study provided evidence that obesity is associated with a higher appearance of heart attacks [14].

The Nurses Health Study involving 115,886 American nurses demonstrated that even a slight increase in the BMI, within the normal range or into the overweight range, dramatically increases the risk for developing diabetes mellitus. Thus, with a body mass index above 30, the risk was about 30 times higher than with a BMI less than 22 [19, 20]. During the course of the 16-year follow-up, an increase in weight of 10–20 kg led to a 20% rise in the total mortality, a 70% increase in cardiovascular mortality, and a 160% increase in coronary heart disease mortality. An average weight increase of 10 kg over 14 years led to a threefold increase in the diabetes incidence, while an increase in weight

Table 3. Co-morbidities and complications of being overweight/obese (based on WHO 2000)

Diabetes mellitus, insulin resistance
Dyslipidemia, low HDL-cholesterol, hypercholesterolemia, hypertriglyceridemia
Coronary heart disease, congestive heart failure, stroke
Cancer, colon-cancer, breast-cancer, endometrial cancer, gallbladder-cancer,
  prostate-cancer, kidney-cancer
Gallstones
Sleep apnea
Osteoarthritis
Increased risk for surgical and anesthetic procedures
Quality of life is reduced, social stigmatization

---

of 11–20 kg led to a fivefold increase. Android fat distribution leads to a higher manifestation of type II diabetes than does the gynoid fat distribution [22].

The high risk of hypercholesteremia – especially of hyper-LDLemia – is clearly defined. Normal cholesterol values are frequently seen with obesity, though a shift in the HDL and LDL concentrations to low HDL and high LDL can be seen [16]. The PROCAM Study presents a prospective investigation of the frequency and the risk character of arteriosclerosis, the classical risk factor. In the PROCAM Study, one likewise sees a clear correlation between triglycerides, for which the risk rating is now clearly defined, and age and body mass index in both genders. The PROCAM Study examined the risk for CHD in 19,682 employees from companies located in Westphalia, Germany [3, 16]. Figure 11 from the PROCAM Study shows the relationship between weight and cardiovascular risk factors, such as hypertension, hypercholesterolemia, hypertriglyceridemia, blood glucose and HDL cholesterol in 17,434 men. A significant increase in the appearance of all risk factors is found with weight gain [3, 16].

The risk of stroke in women having a BMI more than 27 is about 75%; with a BMI above 32, about 137% higher than with a BMI less than 21. Adipose men with android fat distribution are at especially high risk [30]. The sleep apnea syndrome is seen much more frequently among the obese; indeed, more than 80% of all patients with obstructive sleep apnea syndrome are obese. A 4-point increase in the BMI is accompanied by a 4-fold higher risk for sleep-related breathing disorders. Reduction in weight may clearly improve the sleep apnea syndrome [15]. The risk for developing hyperuricemia – as well as of its accompanying disease, gout – rises with the degree of being overweight as the correlation between weight and uric acid concentration is highly significant. The importance of hyperuricemia as a cardiac risk factor is less than the other risk factors [5, 8, 18, 30]. Being overweight or obese also leads to an increase in gallstone formation. In the

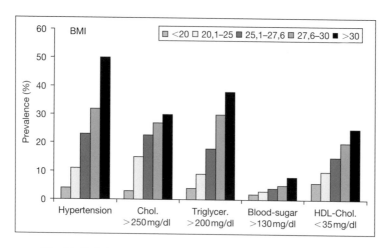

Fig. 11. Relationship between body weight and cardiovascular risk factors. PROCAM Study [3].

Nurses Health Study, women having a body mass index more than 30 had a 2–3 times higher risk for gallstones [19]. With obesity, the excess body weight inevitably leads to increased joint deterioration and to arthroses in knee and hip joints; injury to intervertebral disks is seen more frequently [30].

Increased food ingestion leads to an increased cell metabolism. Increased mitosis rates can result in more errors in mitosis. For this reason, with excessive food ingestion – obesity is always a consequence of increased food ingestion – the incidence of cancer also increases. In women, the risk is particularly increased for endometrial, cervical, and ovarian cancer, as well as for postmenopausal breast cancer; in men, intestinal and prostate cancers are especially seen. The relative risk of dying of cancer is increased by about 55% in adipose women and by about 33% in adipose men [7a] (fig. 12, 13).

Obesity does not present with its own clinical picture of mental disease. It can, however, lead to distinctive psychological disturbances, such as affective and anxiety disorders, as well as depression [4]. Depressions are found twice as frequently among the overweight as among their normal-weight peers. Even though mental disease problems are very frequently seen with obesity, they are, as a rule, not the cause but rather a consequence of being overweight [24, 25].

Among white American women aged 40–64 years, a weight reduction of 10 kg led to a reduction in the total mortality of >20%, a reduction in the diabetes-associated mortality of >30% and to a reduction in the obesity-associated carcinoma mortality by >40% [31]. Weight reduction leads to a significant reduction in the blood pressure, lipid levels, HbA1c and blood glucose [31, 32].

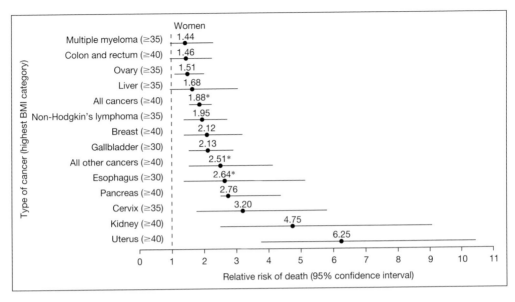

Fig. 12. Summary of mortality from cancer according to body mass index for US women in the Cancer Prevention Study II, 1982 through 1998 [7a].

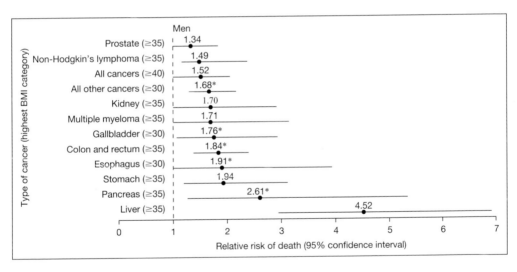

Fig. 13. Summary of mortality from cancer according to body mass index for US men in the Cancer Prevention Study II, 1982 through 1998 [7a].

Being Overweight and Obese Decreases the Quality of Life

The quality of life among the obese is clearly decreased. In a prospective study among women, Fine et al. [9] describe the influences of weight swings on the quality of life. An increase in weight leads to a significant reduction in the quality of life, reduction in weight to an improvement.

The obese are discriminated against socially. In 1971, as queried by a representative survey, some 40% of the population was amenable to accepting an overweight person as their friend; in 1997, only 3% were so inclined. Among the normal weight population, the cause of being overweight is perceived as too much food ingestion by 32%, improper diet by 26%, followed by too little exercise by 11% and heredity by 9%; the overweight see this situation completely differently. Some 17% of obese patients view heredity as the cause, 15% perceive it to be related to a good food conversion ratio (nutrition value of food optimally used), and 20% feel that metabolism, glandular problems, medication or bone structure are responsible. Only 5% indicated that they eat too much and only 22% of the obese perceive the influence of food ingestion in being overweight [9].

Psychological test results show that, when compared to their normal weight counterparts, the overweight have anxiety and depression levels that are 3–4 times higher [4]. The obese classify themselves as socially unattractive. They assume that others talk about them behind their backs. They suffer disadvantages in their professional positions; physicians sometimes treat them disrespectfully.

After successful weight loss, the mental health condition of patients dramatically improves. Among patients who have successfully taken off weight, 90% could more easily imagine accepting an amputated leg or even going blind rather than becoming extremely obese again. These data show that the obese suffer a great psychological burden. Accusations from the so-called 'normal' population also results in obesity being identified as a blameworthy and self-inflicted condition. The disease character is not acknowledged [9, 24].

The psychosocial burden of patients also arises from the fact that the obese are perceived by our social insurance system as being weak, and the health insurance companies deem their being overweight as self-inflicted and brought about by the obese person himself. Occasionally, cost carriers will view this exclusively as a cosmetic-esthetic problem. Great inroads still need to be made in the acceptance and treatment of obesity as a chronic disease.

Somatic and Psychological Consequences among Children and
Adolescents

The appearance of a metabolic syndrome in the overweight and obese almost always occurs, though the latent periods vary greatly. Often, a person is overweight for many years while the consequences of the metabolic syndrome are only seen much later. This is particularly true for the younger organism. Indeed, for many years, no data were available reporting on the development of the metabolic syndrome in young overweight or obese adolescents. Nevertheless, with the dramatic increase in childhood and adolescent obesity, the necessity for clinical and prospective studies arose. These now clearly indicate that even in children and adolescents obesity promotes the development of the metabolic syndrome. In 2004, Weiss and colleagues examined children and adolescents and found that the metabolic syndrome is reported significantly more frequently among today's youths. The prevalence rises directly with the extent of the obesity. A strong correlation was observed between obesity and insulin resistance, as well as C-reactive protein and interleukin-6 levels. In this investigation, the frequency of the metabolic syndrome increased with the extent of being overweight and, in severely obese youths, rose up to 50% [28].

Being Overweight and Obese Decreases the Quality of Life among Children and Adolescents

Even among children and adolescents, the quality of life is clearly decreased when obesity is present. In 2003, Schwimmer and colleagues reported that children and adolescents having a body mass index of 35 scored 67 points on the health-related quality of life scale, while healthy children recorded 83 points. The values for obese children and adolescents were comparable to their peers who had been diagnosed with cancer. Likewise, the quality of life among obese children and adolescents with sleep apnea was, with 54 points, significantly lower than in adipose children and adolescents without sleep apnea. The BMI z score was significantly inversely correlated with the total score, with mental health functioning, social functioning and psychosocial functioning [26].

The authors conclude that obese children and adolescents suffer a lower quality of life than their healthy peers. Obese adolescents are socially discriminated against and are, with respect to their quality of life, comparable with young people in whom cancer has been diagnosed [26].

Conclusion

Being overweight or obese leads to numerous associated diseases that dramatically reduce the quality of life as well as significantly increase morbidity and mortality (fig. 11, 14, 15). Numerous studies prove that being overweight not only leads to the appearance of risk factors for increased mortality, but even considered by itself, also shortens life expectancy.

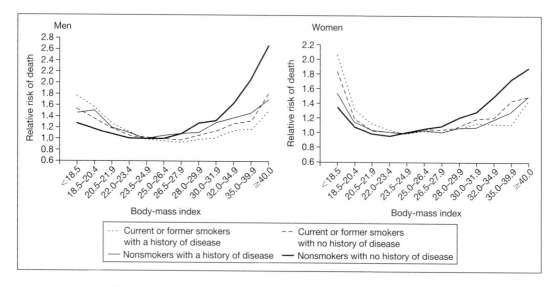

Fig. 14. Multivariate relative risk of death from all causes among men and women according to body mass index, smoking status, and disease status [7b].

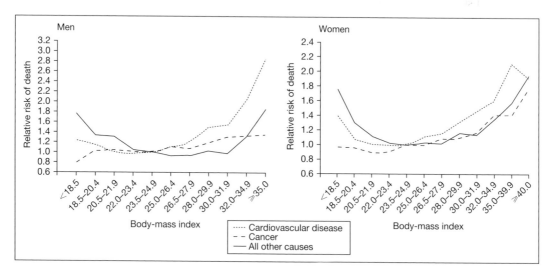

Fig. 15. Multivariate relative risk of death from cardiovascular disease, cancer, and all other causes among men und women who had never smoked and who had no history of disease at enrollment, according to body mass index [7b].

In spite of all therapeutic efforts, the number of people who are overweight and obese is increasing worldwide. This phenomenon is not only the evolutionary-biological command for survival with a genetic optimal ability for storing fat for times of famine, but also the easy availability of food products. In today's world, food ingestion usually occurs very rapidly; food is available in an almost unlimited supply. Therefore, with few exceptions, the energy supply is excessive. An increased energy supply inevitably leads to obesity. Worldwide, enough energy is available for mankind in the form of food. Unfortunately, for political reasons, an equable provision for all populations is not possible. In certain regions of the world, famines appear, while in other areas, a food surplus exists.

In civilized and industrialized countries, obesity prevention is becoming particularly important. Programs must be developed especially for the prevention in childhood and adolescence. Initial attempts seem hopeful, and increasing numbers of government programs are becoming available. Likewise, health insurance companies and insurers are beginning to offer prevention programs.

A multitude of factors contribute to the development of obesity. Consequently, therapy must follow an interdisciplinary and multimodal course. Good short-term, and satisfactory long-term results have been reported from interdisciplinary therapy programs [27]. Accordingly, obesity therapy must continue for at least 12 months and requires medical care, behavioral modification and psychological instruction, training in physical activity as well as nutrition-based information and supervision.

Obesity prevention and obesity therapy must follow defined standards and be in accordance with guidelines from professional societies. Data from the literature demonstrate that weight reduction among the obese and overweight not only lowers the risk factors of arteriosclerosis and associated diseases, but also increases life expectancy [8, 18, 30].

References

1   Arbeitsgemeinschaft Adipositas im Kindes- und Jugendalter (AGA). http://www.a-g-a.de
2   Allison DB, Fontaine KR, Manson JE, Stevens J, VanItalie TB: Annual deaths attributable to obesity in the United States. JAMA 1999;282:1530–1538.
3   Assmann G, Schulte H: Obesity and hyperlipidemia: Results from the Prospective Cardiovascular Munster (PROCAM) Study; in Björntorp P, Brodhoff BN (eds): Obesity. Philadelphia, Lippincott, 1992, pp 502–511.
4   Becker ES, Margraf J, Turke V, et al: Obesity and mental illness in a representative sample of young women. Int J Obes Relat Metab Disord (Engl) 2001;25(suppl 1):S5–S9.
5   Bray GA, Bouchard D, James WPT: Handbook of Obesity. New York, Marcel Dekker, 1998.
6   Bundred P, Kitchiner D, Buchan I: Prevalence of overweight and obese children between 1989 and 1998: Population based series of cross sectional studies. BMJ 2001;322:326–328.

7a   Calle EE, Rodriguez C, Walker-Thurmond K, Thun MJ: Overweight, obesity and mortality from cancer in a prospectively studied cohort of U.S. adults. NEJM 2003;348:1625–1638.

7b   Calle EE, Thun MJ, Petrelli JM, Rodriguez C, Heath CW: Body mass index and mortality in a prospective cohort of US adults. NEJM 1999;341:1097–1105.

8   Clinical Guidelines in the Identification, Evaluation and Treatment of Overweight and Obesity in Adults: National Institute of Health, Washington, 1998, No 6.

9   Fine JT, Colditz GA, Coakley EH, et al: A prospective study of weight change and health-related quality of life in women. JAMA 1999;282:2136–2142.

10   Flegal KM: Prevalence and trends in obesity among US adults, 1999–2000. JAMA 2002;288: 1723–1727.

11   Fontaine KR, Redden DT, Wang C, Westfall AO, Allison DB: Years of life lost due to obesity. JAMA 2003;289:187–193.

12   Gesundheitsberichterstattung des Bundes, Heft 16, Übergewicht und Adipositas, Robert-Koch-Institut, Statistisches Bundesamt, 2003.

13   Hedley AA, Ogden CL, Johnson CL, Carroll MD, Curtin LR, Flegal KM: Prevalence of over-weight und obesity among US children, adolescents and adults, 1999–2002. JAMA 2004;291: 2847–2850.

14   Hubert HB, Feinlieb M, McNamara PM, Castelli WP: Obesity as an independent risk factor for cardiovascular disease: A 26 year follow-up of participants in the Framing-ham heart study. Circulation 1983;67:968–977.

15   Kansanen M, Vanninen E, Tuunainen A, Pesonen P: The effect of a very low-calorie diet-induced weight loss on the severity of obstructive sleep apnoea and autonomic nervous function in obese patients with obstructive sleep apnoea syndrome. Clin Physiol 1998;18:377–385.

16   Klose G: Adipositas und Hyperlipidämie. Adipositas – Ursachen und Therapie. Berlin, JG Wechsler, Blackwell, 2003, pp 175–193.

17   Lakka HM, Laaksonen DE, Lakka TA, Niskanen LK, Kumpusalo E, Tuomilehto J, Salonen JT: The metabolic syndrome and total and cardiovascular disease mortality in middle-aged men. JAMA 2002;288:2709–2716.

18   Leitlinien der Deutschen Adipositas-Gesellschaft zur Therapie der Adipositas. Adipositas II, 1998.

19   Manson JE, Willett WC, Stapfer MJ, Colditz GA, Hunter DJ, Hankinson SE, Hennekens CH, Speizer FE: Body weight and mortality among women. NEJM 1995;333:677–685.

20   Manson JE, Rimm EB, Stampfer MJ, Colditz JA, Willett WC, Krolewski AS, Rossner B, Hennekens CH, Speizer FE: Physical activity and incidence of non-insulin-dependent diabetes mellitus in women. Lancet 1991;338:774–778.

21   Mokdad AH, Serdula MK, Dietz WH, et al: The spread of the obesity epidemic in the United States, 1991–1998. JAMA 1999;282:1519–1522.

22   Mokdad AH, Ford ES, Bowman BA, Dietz WH, Vinicor F, Bales VS, Marks JS: Prevalence of obesity, diabetes, and obesity-related health risk factors, 2001. JAMA 2003;298:76–79.

23   Ogden CL: Prevalence and trends in overweight among US children and adolescents, 1999–2000. JAMA 2002;288:1728–1732.

24   Pudel V: Psychologische Ansätze in der Adipositas-Therapie. Bundesgesundheitsblatt. Gesundheitsforschung – Gesundheitsschutz 10, 2001, pp 954–959.

25   Rexrode KM, Hennekens CH, Willet WC, Colditz GA, Stampfer MJ, Rich-Edwards JW, Speizer FE, Manson JE: A prospective study of body mass index, weight change, and risk of stroke in women. JAMA 1997;277:1539–1545.

26   Schwimmer JB, Burwinkle TM, Varni JW: Health-related quality of life of severely obese children and adolescents. JAMA 2003;289:1813–1819.

27   Wechsler JG (Hrsg.): Adipositas – Ursachen und Therapie. Wien/Berlin, Blackwell-Verlag, 2003.

28   Weiss R, Dziura J, Burgert TS, Tamborlane WV, Taksali SE, Yeckel CW, Allen K, Lopes M, Savoye M, Morrison J, Sherwin RS, Caprio S: Obesity and the metabolic syndrome in children and adolescents. NEJM 2004;350:2362–2374.

29   Wenzel H: Definition, Klassifikation und Messung der Adipositas; in Wechsler JG (Hrsg.): 'Adipositas'. Berlin, Blackwell-Verlag, 2003, pp 47–63.

30   WHO-Report Obesity: Preventing and managing the global epidemic. WHO, Geneva, 2000.

31 Williamson DF, Pamuk E, Thun M, Flanders D, Byers T, Heath C: Prospective study of intentional weight loss and mortality in never-smoking overweight US white women aged 40–64 years. Am J Epidemiol 1995;141:1128–1141.
32 Williamson DF, Thompson TJ, Thun M, Flanders D, Pamuk E, Byers T: Intentional weight loss and mortality among overweight individuals with diabetes. Diabetes Care 2000;23:1499–1504.

Prof. Dr. med. J.G. Wechsler
Krankenhaus Barmherzige Brüder, Innere Abteilung
Romanstrasse 93, DE–80639 München (Germany)
Tel. +49 89 1797 2401, Fax +49 89 1797 2420
E-Mail prof.wechsler@barmherzige-muenchen.de

Munsch S, Beglinger C (eds): Obesity and Binge Eating Disorder.
Bibl Psychiatr. Basel, Karger, 2005, No 171, pp 62–73

Etiology of Obesity

Claus Vögele

School of Psychology and Therapeutic Studies,
Roehampton University, London, UK

Etiology of Obesity

Determining the causes of obesity is central to any efforts to tackling it. However, despite years of research uncertainty over the etiology of obesity remains one of the chief barriers to designing effective strategies for prevention and treatment [1]. Many studies have been carried out into the potential influence of genetic factors, such as possible metabolic defects, and these have yielded promising results in identifying gene mutations that render affected individuals predisposed to develop obesity. However, this has been shown only for a small percentage of morbidly obese patients, and it is unlikely that there is a single genetic cause in the majority of cases. This is particularly true as the dramatically escalating rate of obesity documented in recent years has occurred in a relatively constant gene pool.

Important as these advances in our knowledge of the genetic basis of obesity are, they tend to obscure the obvious: that genetic susceptibility will rarely cause obesity in the absence of 'obesogenic' environmental factors.

At its simplest level, obesity is caused when energy intake exceeds energy expenditure. This seemingly straightforward equation is, however, complicated by a multitude of factors impacting upon this delicate balance. At the level of energy intake eating behaviors and related psychological and physiological processes of hunger and satiety regulation are crucial. At the level of energy expenditure reduced physical activity, lower thermogenesis, i.e. smaller increases in metabolic rate in response to food intake, and an overall reduction in resting metabolic rate are all likely to contribute to a chronic positive energy imbalance between energy intake and energy expenditure.

Most accounts of the shifts in obesity prevalence over time draw not on changes in social or psychological conditions, but on the combination of an environment which favors a positive energy balance and an appetite control system which evolved when the food supply was limited. There is now an abundant, highly palatable, food supply in industrialized countries. At the same time, transportation systems and mechanization have reduced the energy demands of everyday life. If human beings evolved to store energy supplies, then it is not surprising that so many people are now overweight [2]. While this evolutionary perspective might serve to explain the increase in prevalence rates on a population level, it does not explain why some people are so much fatter than others, why some preserve a stable body weight or indeed, why others succeed in maintaining a low body weight when everyone else finds it so difficult. This chapter will give an overview of genetic and environmental factors currently thought to contribute to the development of obesity.

Genetic Factors

The frequently made observation that obesity tends to run in families is now supported by both molecular genetics and genetic epidemiology. Results from molecular genetic investigations show that monogenic forms of extreme obesity are associated with mutations of the melanocortin-4-receptor (Mc4r) [3]. This, however, is true only for 3–5% of all morbidly obese individuals (BMI $\geq$40). Not all individuals, however, with this Mc4r mutation are obese suggesting that obesity may depend on genetic variation in other genes in these individuals. In the vast majority of cases it is assumed that a multitude of genes are involved in processes that affect body fatness, e.g. energy intake, energy expenditure and partitioning (i.e. storage of calories in fat, glycogen and proteins).

Heritability of obesity, i.e. the fraction of the population variation in obesity that can be explained by genetic transmission, has been considered in a large number of twin, adoption and family studies. Heritability levels for identical twins, fraternal twins or twins reared apart tend to cluster around 70% of the variation in BMI. In contrast, adoption studies have generated the lowest heritability estimates of 30% or less. Heritability levels from family studies are reported to fall in between these latter two categories. There is controversy over the interpretation of these results with some seeing them as strong evidence for the role of genetic factors in the etiology of obesity. Others conclude that the heritability level reaches about one-third of the population variance, and that changes in lifestyle account for the major part of the variance.

Another way of studying the genetics of obesity is through quantifying the risk of becoming obese when a first-degree relative is overweight or obese. Recently reported results show that although the prevalence of obesity is twice as high in families of obese individuals as in the general population at large, this effect is dependent on the severity of obesity. Katzmarzyk et al. [4], for example, showed that the familial risk of obesity was five times higher for relatives in the upper 1% of the distribution of BMI values than in the general population. The results also suggested that the risk of becoming obese was not entirely due to genetic factors as the risk was also elevated in cohabitating spouses of study participants. This latter result in particular suggests a complex genotype-environment interaction where the response of a phenotype to environmental changes such as diet or physical activity levels depends on the genotype of the individual. Intervention trials have shown considerable interindividual differences in the response to various dietary interventions or exercise programs. Studies with identical twins, for example, revealed that the response to positive or negative energy balance is very heterogeneous between twin pairs but quite homogeneous within members of the same twin pair [5].

In summary, important advances have been made in the genetics of obesity albeit we are still only beginning to understand the basis of complex gene-gene and gene-environment interactions. The identification of genes associated with the etiology of obesity is a difficult task in familial or pedigree studies. Whatever the impact of the genotype on the etiology of obesity, it is generally attenuated or exacerbated by non-genetic, environmental factors, particularly in the presence of an obesogenic environment.

The dramatically escalating rate of obesity documented in recent years is often quoted as an indication of the dominant role of environmental factors as these changes have occurred in a relatively constant gene pool. In fact, this situation only highlights the importance of distinguishing between genes causing obesity from those predisposing to it. Significant advances have been made in the identification of the former although they may account for only a small percentage of all obesity cases. It is the identification of the latter that poses the daunting task of defining how genetic individuality interacts with the environment to make some people resistant to obesity and others very much at risk to becoming obese [6].

Prenatal Factors

A further example of gene-environment interactions – however, at a very early point in life – comes from studies investigating the effects of the in utero environment and later disease or metabolic functioning [7]. Extreme caloric deprivation during critical periods in pregnancy and a resulting low birth weight is positively associated with a higher than average weight during childhood and also later in life [8]. Higher birth weight has also been linked to greater likelihood of being obese early in childhood. Children born to mothers with insulin-dependent diabetes are at greater risk for being overweight, even after controlling for maternal weight.

These observations have been also subsumed in the literature under the term 'metabolic programming' or 'fetal priming'. This notion suggests that the environment in utero can affect the metabolic phenotype as a form of metabolic programming. The in utero environment does not change the genes of the individual; it changes the way the genes are expressed, either in utero or later in life.

An example for the processes that are involved in fetal priming comes from cardiovascular research [9]. Low birth weight (indicating fetal malnutrition) has been shown to be associated with an increased risk for essential hypertension in later life. Fetal priming models assume that the fetus – if it experiences malnutrition – expresses genes that lead to the production of vasoconstricting hormones. This not only leads to a better blood supply through the placenta but will also raise maternal blood pressure (pre-eclampsia). Expression of these genes later in life, re-activated through the effects of environmental factors, may lead to established essential hypertension. The proposed mechanisms involved in the fetal priming of obesity include effects of maternal insulin levels on the development of the fetal pancreas and more generally permanent adaptations of central regulatory mechanisms of energy intake and expenditure.

These results serve to highlight the fact that gene-environment interactions begin much earlier in life than previously thought, i.e. in the womb. In summary, the current literature suggests that a birth weight at either end of the distribution, i.e. lower or higher than average, increases the risk for later obesity (and a range of other disorders). The underlying metabolic processes might be quite varied, but they all seem to impact on future regulation of energy balance and body weight.

However, although a predisposition towards obesity may be 'written in the genes', it is not indelible. The inclination is to some degree alterable during various periods of life: prenatally through avoiding malnutrition or maternal obesity or diabetes, but also in early childhood and into adolescence. As children age, this window of plasticity may start to close. It is evident from this brief account of prenatal gene-environment interactions that early interventions are important. We have argued elsewhere that food preferences are acquired in childhood and sound nutritional practices should therefore be established in childhood as a basis for life-long healthy eating [10]. In the context of the findings on fetal programming it seems such interventions should be extended to include the prenatal period by ensuring adequate maternal nutrition.

Dietary Habits

The advances in understanding the genetic basis of obesity are also psychologically important. They show that the often made causal attributions of individuals of 'their' obesity to genetic or biological determinants (e.g. 'I am just making proper use of the food I eat') do not lack empirical support all together. However, at the level of energy intake there is increasing evidence that it is not only important *how much* we eat but also *what* we eat. Large-scale investigations over the last 10 years, for example, have shown that the so-called carbohydrate fattening, i.e. the lipogenesis from carbohydrates, does not represent a major metabolic route in the development of obesity [11]. In contrast to other species, in humans carbohydrates are converted to fat only after several days' consumption of more than 500 g of carbohydrates per day. This amount is roughly equivalent to 500 g sugar, 1.2 kg of bread, 3 kg of pasta, 3.5 kg of potatoes or 30 kg of cauliflower. Several field studies of large cohorts have shown a positive linear relationship between body weight and fat consumption, but a negative correlation with carbohydrate intake [12]. With calories from fat accounting for more than 46% of daily calorific consumption obese individuals consume relatively more calories from fat than from carbohydrates; this is significantly more than the recommended 30% for the general population [13, 14]. These results are in conflict with previous weight reduction interventions which tend to reduce calorific intake irrespective of macronutrient source. As body fat is primarily generated from dietary fat, but not from carbohydrates, the dietary fat preference of many overweight and obese individuals represents an important etiological factor and has far reaching implications for weight reduction interventions.

Eating Behavior

As discussed earlier obesity is the result of energy intake exceeding energy expenditure, or – put in a more simple way – if one eats more than one needs. Psychologists' first incursions into understanding why people eat too much focused on psychodynamically orientated models suggesting that eating too much served unconscious needs and that levels of psychopathology are, therefore, higher than in the normal-weight population. Empirical findings from studies investigating the prevalence of mental disorders in obese individuals do not support this latter assumption, although there is evidence that severely obese individuals have raised levels of depression and anxiety. This, however, appears to be an effect rather than a cause of obesity, strongly associated with the experience of multiple handicaps and stigmatization [15, 16].

Cognitive theories of eating behavior stipulate differences in the experience of hunger and satiety and, therefore, in the regulation of eating behavior. Schachter's [17] externality model suggests that obesity is caused by low responsiveness to internal cues for satiety combined with high responsiveness to external food cues. Results from laboratory studies showed differences in responsiveness to food between obese and normal-weight adults, and the theory was further supported by observations on animal models of obesity. Despite these initial successes subsequent studies failed to replicate the major findings [18]. Former students of Schachter put forward their own theories in order to explain some of the inconsistencies: Nisbett's set point theory [19] and Herman and Polivy's concept of restraint eating and the boundary model [20]. Common to both theories is the assumption that the crucial factor mediating the association between obesity and externality is not obesity per se but the constant dieting behavior which is the result of social pressures to be slim. According to the more biological set point-theory each individual has a set level of fat stores which are defended by up-regulating appetite if they are depleted and down-regulated if they are filled. Obese people were thought to have a higher than normal set-point, resulting in abnormal appetite if they lost weight below their own set point weight.

Despite its clear simplicity this theory has been largely abandoned as it cannot, for example, explain the shift in set-point weights over the last decade given the recent increase in obesity prevalence. At the core of Herman and Polivy's boundary model [20] lies the assumption that dieting behavior annuls normal hunger and satiety regulation through suppression of internal cues, and replaces it with cognitive control mechanisms, i.e. dietary restraint. By trying to eat less than they would otherwise want to, dieting obese individuals, according to this model, have 'unlearned' to respond to their internal signals of hunger and satiety [see also chapter on childhood obesity by Braet, pp. 117–137].

This system of deliberate control over eating requires an almost permanent conscious effort in order maintain it. It is, therefore, easy to perturb: both any kind of distraction (e.g. strong emotions) and breaking the dietary rule (e.g. by eating 'forbidden' food) have been shown to lead to loss of control over eating and in some instances even to binge eating. There is now considerable evidence that restrained eaters are less responsive to satiety, more responsive to palatability, and more likely to show over-eating in response to negative affect. Recent results [21, 22] have further added to and differentiated this picture: restraint per se does not seem to predict overeating in an experimental situation; it is the tendency to over-eat – in combination with restraint – that is crucial in eliciting overeating and binge eating. The individuals most at risk are not those who are restraint but do not over eat; they might well be described as successful dieters. It is those who show the combination of high restraint and a high tendency to overeat, therefore having susceptibility toward failure of restraint.

These observations turned existing ideas on their head in suggesting that attempts to regulate food intake (in combination with a tendency to over eat) might be the cause of, and not simply a response to, problems of eating control. By logical extension they also suggest that previous intervention approaches to control body weight by prescribing calorie reduced diets may actually contribute to the problem of obesity and not solve it. The observation that up to 85% of participants in weight loss programs based on calorific reduction alone regain their initial weight and more over a period of five years after the end of the program lends some support to this notion [23].

The association between restraint and regulatory problems is now well established, but there is still uncertainty about the mechanism, and especially about why restrained eaters should ever actually eat *more* than unrestrained eaters. The cognitive model of restraint proposes that after a high calorie pre-load (in the laboratory) or a dieting transgression (in everyday life), the dieter 'reasons' that she might as well take advantage of the situation and leave dieting until tomorrow. The psycho-biological model suggests that after a long history of imposed cognitive control, in which normal biological controls have been over-ridden and food intake patterns are chaotic and irregular, sensitivity to satiety or hunger signals becomes blunted and learned patterns of hunger and satiety are disrupted. The emotional model suggests that the dieter copes with negative emotional states with dissociation, and as part of this, loses contact with her restrictive intentions. There is some evidence for each of these processes, but as yet there have been no definitive studies which distinguish between them.

It seems likely that restraint can increase the risk of loss of control, but there may be riskier and less risky forms. Flexible restraint has been associated with better weight control than rigid restraint. Eating regimens with regular meal patterns and a balanced nutrient intake are probably better than short-term drastic restriction. Negative body image is very often the motive for attempts at weight loss, but may in itself increase the difficulty of controlling weight, so interventions which improve body image could facilitate weight control. Higher levels of physical exercise are consistently associated with better weight control, both in the normal population and in maintaining weight loss after treatment, and deserve a higher profile in psychological treatments.

Physical (In)Activity

Given the current rise in obesity prevalence, it may come as a surprise that the average level of energy intake has actually fallen in western countries since the 1960s [24]. This apparent contradiction can only be explained if the average level of energy input is falling more slowly than the average level of energy output, thus creating the conditions for increases in average weight levels and prevalence of obesity.

There is no doubt that people living in today's societies are less physically active than they have probably ever been in history. Although measuring activity levels is difficult because they usually rely on self-report measures, recent national surveys [e.g. 25] and reports by the WHO [26] conclude that the extra physical activity involved in living 50 years ago, compared to today was the equivalent to running a marathon a week. So why have lifestyles changed so dramatically over the last 50 years? A first answer lies in the increasing use of motorized transport instead of active methods of transport, such as walking and cycling. The latest UK National Travel Survey [27] indicates that the average person now walks 189 miles per year, a fall of 66 miles over 25 years. This decline in walking may be attributed to the loss of opportunities to walk, as well as increased access to motorized transport. The increasing use of cars has led to a vicious circle of car dependency, as town planning has increasingly prioritized the needs of motorists above those of pedestrians and cyclists, meaning that in many places walking and cycling are at best unpleasant and at worst dangerous. At the same time, local neighborhoods are increasingly perceived by parents as unsafe for children to play out in, implicitly discouraging active play and contributing to the growing problem of physical inactivity in children.

Activity levels for children appear to have fallen in almost every aspect of their lives. The recent Chief Medical Officer's report suggested that 2 in 10 boys and girls undertake less than 30 min activity a day [28]. According to the organization Working for Cycling, in 1985–1986 only 22% of 5- to 10-year-olds were driven to school; that figure had risen to 39% by 1999–2000. Some schools are reported to have even put seats in playground areas so that children can sit for the whole of their lunch break.

Television viewing is another factor contributing to the current levels of inactivity: the average person in the 1960s watched television 13 h a week compared to 26 h now [29]. Gortmaker et al. [30] have shown that adolescents spending more than 5 hours per day with television viewing are 4.6 times more likely to be obese than those with a television consumption of 2 h or less.

Results from cross-sectional comparisons of physical activity levels between obese and normal-weight individuals are equivocal. This has a number of methodological and conceptual reasons. Studies have, for example, used a variety of different measures to quantify energy expenditure. They range from highly sophisticated laboratory methods with very good reliability and extremely poor ecological validity to self-report data where the relation between reliability and validity is reversed. Conceptual problems in defining what constitutes physical activity are another example, which makes direct comparisons between studies all but impossible. Investigations have considered the entire armory of physical activity behavior ranging from micro movements to everyday activities and exercise, however not combined in one study making it difficult to arrive at firm conclusions about physical activity level differences in general. Finally, only few studies take into consideration that obese individuals use more calories when physically active than their normal weight counterparts as they have to move more body weight; this is very frequently overlooked in drawing direct comparisons between activity levels of obese and normal weight individuals.

In summary, there is evidence that physical activity levels have declined dramatically over the last few decades in the general population and this coincides with a rise in the prevalence of obesity. Extraordinary as these findings are it has to be said that they only provide incidental and correlational evidence for the role of inactivity in the etiology of obesity. To our knowledge no study has shown a direct causal route of inactivity that leads to obesity, nor do we know the differential impact of lack of physical activity in the energy balance equation. Cross-sectional comparisons of physical activity levels between obese and normal weight individuals do not contribute to the clarification of these questions either as they suffer from methodological heterogeneity and a lack of conceptual clarity. Moreover, given their cross-sectional design only tentative conclusions about a causal role of lack of physical activity could be drawn.

Notwithstanding these methodological criticisms the findings on the decline of physical activity levels on a population level are impressive still, particularly as sedentary behavior has been shown to be a significant risk factor for a range of diseases other than obesity. There is also evidence that some of the health benefits associated with increased levels of physical activity are in fact independent of weight loss (e.g. improvements in cardio-respiratory fitness and blood lipid profiles, reductions in plasma-insulin concentrations and increased insulin sensitivity) [31].

There is now an impressive body of literature confirming the benefits of regular physical activity for both physical and mental health [32]. The American Centers for Disease Control and Prevention and the American College of Sports Medicine concluded in a joint report that evidence from cross sectional epidemiological surveys as well as controlled, experimental studies suggests that physically active adults tend to develop and maintain better physical health [33]. The report further concludes that prolonged vigorous exercise is not necessary to achieve these benefits and recommends an increase in everyday physical activity amounting to a total of at least 30 min activity at an intensity corresponding to brisk walking. This activity level should be well within the grasp of most people. It is puzzling, therefore, that physical activity levels in the general population are well below this recommended intensity and drop-out rates from exercise programs continue to be high, particularly amongst those who would benefit most (i.e. cardiac patients, obese individuals). Data from Europe and the USA suggests that the majority of people start to exercise at one point during their lives, but only a minority succeeds in turning this behavior into a lifelong habit. Low levels of physical activity in the general population are, therefore, not so much a consequence of a lack of motivation to start but a result of difficulties to maintain exercise behavior. This clearly has important implications for the design of therapeutic interventions to increase physical activity levels.

Conclusions

Obesity is likely to be caused by complex gene-gene and gene-environment interactions. Despite significant advances in the understanding of the genetics of obesity, a genetic predisposition for obesity is generally exacerbated by non-genetic, environmental factors. There is increasing evidence that the prenatal (in utero) environment plays an important role in affecting adaptations of central regulatory mechanisms of energy intake and expenditure, thus potentially increasing the risk for obesity later in life. As obesity is caused when energy intake exceeds energy expenditure over-eating is a significant etiological factor. Psychological investigations of over-eating have identified a cognitive-behavioral pattern characterized by deliberate but unsuccessful control over eating as a significant risk factor for problems with food intake regulation. However, for the etiology of obesity it is not only important *how much* we eat but also *what* we eat: There is a positive association between body weight and fat consumption, but a negative correlation with carbohydrate intake. As body fat is primarily generated from dietary fat, but not from carbohydrates, the dietary fat preference of many overweight and obese individuals represents an important etiological factor and has far reaching implications for weight reduction interventions. Lack of regular physical exercise is also a major determinant of weight gain and obesity. There is evidence that physical activity levels have declined dramatically over the last few decades in the general population and this coincides with a rise in the prevalence of obesity. This is even more worrying as sedentary behavior has been shown to be a significant risk factor not only for obesity but also a whole range of other diseases. The majority of people start to exercise at one point during their lives, but only a minority succeeds in turning this behavior into a lifelong habit. Low levels of physical activity in the general population are, therefore, not so much a consequence of a lack of motivation to start but a result of difficulties to maintain an active life style. This has important implications for the design of therapeutic interventions to increase physical activity levels.

References

1   Jebb S, Prentice A: Obesity in Britain: Gluttony or sloth? BMJ 1995;311:437–439.
2   Hill JO, Peters JC: Environmental contributions to the obesity epidemic. Science 1998;280: 1371–1374.
3   Yeo GS, Farooqi IS, Aminian S, Halsall DJ, Stanhope RG, O'Rahilly S: A frameshift mutation in MC4R associated with dominantly inherited human obesity. Nat Genet 1998;20:111–112.
4   Katzmarzyk PT, Perusse L, Rao DC, Bouchard C: Familial risk of obesity and central adipose tissue distribution in the general Canadian population. Am J Epidemiol 1999;149:933–942.
5   Bouchard C: Genetic and energy balance interactions in humans; in Bernadier CD (ed): Nutrients and Gene Expression: Clinical Aspects. Boca Raton, CRC Press, 1996, pp 83–100.
6   Barsh GS, Farooqi I, O'Rahilly S: Genetics of body-weight regulation. Nature 2000;404:644–651.
7   Barker DJ, Gluckman PD, Godfrey KM, Harding JE, Owens JA, Robinson JS: Fetal nutrition and cardiovascular disease in adult life. Lancet 1993;341:938–941.
8   Ravelli AC, van Der Meulen JH, Osmond C, Barker DJ, Bleker OP: Obesity at the age of 50 in men and women exposed to famine prenatally. Am J Clin Nutr 1999;70:811–816.
9   Haig D: Genetic conflicts in human pregnancy. Q Rev Biol 1993;68:495–532.
10 Vögele C: Education; in Kerr J, Weitkunat R, Moretti M (eds): The ABC of Behavior Change. Edinburgh, Elsevier, 2004, pp 271–287.
11 Horton TJ, Drougas H, Brachey A, Reed GW, Peters JC, Hill JO: Fat and carbohydrate overfeeding in humans: Different effects on energy storage. Am J Clin Nutr 1995;62:19–29.
12 Bolton-Smith C, Woodward M: Dietary composition and fat to sugar ratios in relation to obesity. Int J Obes 1994;18:820–828.
13 Deutsche Gesellschaft für Ernährung: Empfehlungen für die Nährstoffzufuhr. 5. Korrigierte Überarbeitung. Frankfurt/Main, Umschau Verlag, 1995.
14 Department of Health and Human Services, Department of Agriculture: Nutrition and your Health: Dietary Guidelines for Americans, ed 5. Washington, 2000.
15 Becker ES, Margraf J, Turke V, Soeder U, Neumer S: Obesity and mental illness in a representative sample of young women. Int J Obes 2001;25(suppl 1):S5–S9.
16 Sobal J: Obesity and nutritional sociology: A model for coping with the stigma of obesity. Clin Sociol Rev 1991;9:125–141.
17 Schachter S: Emotion, Obesity, and Crime. New York, Academic Press, 1971.
18 Rodin J: Current status of the internal-external hypothesis for obesity. Am Psychol 1981; 36:361–372.
19 Nisbett RE: Hunger, obesity, and the ventromedial hypothalamus. Psychol Rev 1972;79:433–453.
20 Herman CP, Polivy J: A boundary model for the regulation of eating; in Stunkard JA, Stellar E (eds): Eating and Its Disorders. New York, Raven Press, 1984, pp 141–156.
21 van Strien T, Cleven A, Schippers G: Restraint, tendency toward overeating and ice cream consumption. Int J Eat Disord 2000;28:333–338.
22 Ouwens MA, van Strien T, van der Staak CPF: Tendency toward overeating and restraint as predictors of food consumption. Appetite 2003;40:291–298.
23 Ayyad C, Andersen T: Long-term efficacy of dietary treatment of obesity: A systematic review of studies published between 1931 and 1999. Obes Rev 2000;1:113–119.
24 Webb GP: Nutrition: A Health Promotion Approach. London, Arnold, 1995.
25 National Audit Office: Tackling obesity in England. Report by the comptroller and auditor general HC 220, 2001.
26 World Health Organization: Obesity: Preventing and Managing the Global Epidemic. Report of WHO Consultation on Obesity. Geneva, World Health Organization, 1998.
27 Department for Transport: Transport trends: current edition. http://www.dft.gov.uk/stellent/ groups/dft_transstats/documents/page/dft_transstats_508294.hcsp.
28 Department of Health, Chief Medical Officer: At least five a week: Evidence on the impact of physical activity and its relationship to health, 2004.
29 Office of Population Census and Surveys: General Household Survey. London, Her Majesty's Stationery Office, 1994.

30 Gortmaker StL, Must A, Sobol AM, Peterson K, Colditz CA, Dietz WH: Television viewing as a cause on increasing obesity among children in the United States, 1986–1990. Arch Pediatr Adol Med 1996;150:356–362.

31 Vögele C: Sport und Bewegung als Behandlungsansatz [Exercise and physical activity in the treatment of obesity]; in Petermann F, Pudel V (eds): Adipositas. Göttingen, Hogrefe, 2003, pp 283–302.

32 Astrand PO: Why exercise? Med Sci Sports Exer 1992;24:153–162.

33 Pate RR, Pratt M, Blair SN, Haskell WL, Macera CA, Bouchard C, Buchner D, Ettinger W, Heath GW, King AC, et al: Physical activity and public health: A recommendation from the Centers for Disease Control and the American College of Sports Medicine. JAMA 1995;273:402–407.

Prof. Dr. Claus Vögele
School of Psychology and Therapeutic Studies
Roehampton University, London SW15 3SN (UK)
Tel. +44 0 20 8392 3510, Fax +44 0 20 8394 3610, E-Mail C.Vogele@Roehampton.ac.uk

Munsch S, Beglinger C (eds): Obesity and Binge Eating Disorder.
Bibl Psychiatr. Basel, Karger, 2005, No 171, pp 74–80

....

Treatment Options of Obesity: Behavioral Weight Control

Reinhold G. Laessle

University of Trier, Research Department, Clinical Psychology
of Nutrition, Trier, Germany

The principles and application of behavior therapy for obesity are outlined. The specific features of the behavioral approach for obesity are: goal orientation, direct modification of eating and exercise behavior, process orientation and evaluation, and the advocation of small rather than large changes. The major treatment components consist of self-monitoring, stimulus control techniques, cognitive restructuring, problem solving, nutritional education, and increasing the amount of physical activity. Short-term data on effectiveness of behavioral treatment indicate a very favorable outcome with weight losses of about 10% of initial weight. Further research should address long-term efficacy and strategies to maintain the successful initial weight loss.

The application of behavior therapy to obesity began in the late 1960s with Stuart's [1] case report of the highly successful treatment of 8 individuals who lost an average of 18 kg, a loss of the size of which was achieved by fewer than 5% of persons who received the conventional dietary therapy. The behavioral approach of Stuart was founded on his belief that 'only two common characteristics have been observed in obese persons: a tendency to overeat and a tendency to underexercise'. This statement clearly reflects an oversimplification of the etiology of obesity. Nevertheless, the majority of behaviorally oriented interventions for obesity try to modify energy intake, energy expenditure or both.

Behavior therapy of obesity is based on the functional analysis of behavior [i.e. 2]. Eating and exercise habits are analyzed to determine their relationship to other events including times, places, emotions, cognitions, and other persons. The behavioral approach can be characterized by the following features: (1) It is goal oriented. The objectives of therapy are clearly defined and specified in terms that can be easily measured. (2) Treatment seeks to directly change behavior, which is at present likely to maintain the overweight. Thus, it differs from dynamically oriented therapy, which for example would explore unconscious drives to overeat rooting back to early childhood. (3) Behavioral treatment is process oriented. It is more than helping people decide *what* they want to accomplish; it helps them identify *how* to do so. Patients are encouraged to identify the specific behavior they wish to adopt and when, where, and with whom they will practice it. In cases in which the behavior is not adopted, attention is focused to find alternative strategies. This skill-building philosophy views weight management as a set of skills to be learned rather than as willpower to be enhanced. (4) Behavioral approaches advocate small rather than large changes. This method is based on the learning principle of successive approximation in which incremental steps are taken to achieve more distant goals. Making small changes gives patients successful experiences upon which to build, rather than attempting drastic changes, which are typically short-lived.

In most cases behavioral treatments are offered as multimodal treatment packages. These packages are designed for inpatient as well as for outpatient treatment.

In the following, the major components of treatment are described and illustrated by examples of intervention.

Initial Evaluation and Goals of Treatment

During the initial evaluation the therapist has to collect information on the patient's current social functioning, on the individual's understanding of his or her weight problem, and on the reasons why the patient has sought treatment. Biological factors and genetics, which may contribute to the patient's obesity, should be taken into account additionally. Of great importance is information concerning eating, exercise, and dietary habits, which will be used to plan treatment [3]. Behavioral treatment not only has goals in terms of weight loss but also goals with respect to psychosocial changes. The selection of a reasonable goal weight should be based on the patient's weight history. As a general rule, the goal weight should be no lower than the patient's lowest weight since age 21, which was maintained for at least 1 year [4]. In most cases, an initial weight loss of 10% is sufficient to improve medical complications such as hypertension, diabetes, or hypercholesterolemia. Patient and therapist must explicitly discuss the patient's desired weight loss and the rapidity with which it is anticipated. In the absence of such a discussion, patients frequently adhere to their often unrealistic goals and become treatment dropouts, when they fail to reach them [5].

There is little likelihood that psychosocial benefits will result by weight loss alone. Weight loss may be a necessary condition for such changes, but rarely is it sufficient. Therefore concrete treatment goals should be set in all areas of social functioning (e.g. communication, work, family, self-assertiveness).

Treatment Components

Self-Monitoring

Self-monitoring (observing and recording one's behavior) is a cornerstone of behavioral treatment. Patients are asked to record daily the types and amounts of food that they eat and their caloric value. This practice helps to identify problem foods and hidden sources of calories, and facilitates adherence to a reduced calorie diet. Record keeping is expanded over time to include information on exercise habits, as well as times, places, and feelings associated with eating. In the later stages of treatment, patients attempt to identify high-risk situations that are associated with dietary lapses and record their thoughts and feelings in response to such occurrences. Patients discuss in weekly sessions their success in completing their records and receive feedback from the therapist on methods in handling any problems. Many patients come to view self-monitoring as the most important part of their behavioral programme, and it vastly increases their awareness of their eating behavior.

Stimulus Control

Stimulus control techniques are designed to limit the individual's exposure to food and thus prevent incidental eating. The main assumption is that all stimuli which might be related to the consumption of food should be arranged so as to become antecedents of an adequate eating behavior [2]. This strategy includes the following procedures: (a) Shopping carefully to keep problem foods out of the home (for example with a prescribed shopping list). (b) Storing foods out of sight. (c) Leaving food on the plate and to eliminate it directly into the trash container, when eating is finished. (d) Limiting the times, places and activities associated with eating (e.g. eating three meals a day at a table in the same room without reading or looking television).

Positive cues are used to increase physical activity. These cues might include placing a treadmill in a frequently used room, leaving walking shoes at the front door, or keeping an activity calendar on the refrigerator.

Both self-monitoring as well as stimulus control has empirically been found effective [6].

Cognitive Restructuring

Cognitive therapy is designed to help dieters overcome self-defeating thoughts, which undermine weight control efforts. Such thoughts might include:
- the impossibility of weight loss ('I'll never be able to lose this weight')
- unrealistic goals ('I'll never eat ice cream again')
- self-disparaging statements ('what a failure, I'll always be fat').

Patients identify their negative thoughts through self-monitoring and role-play their rational responses to them.

Methods developed by Beck are used to help patients establish coping-oriented, rational responses to their negativistic beliefs.

Cooper et al. [7] have proposed the use of cognitive therapy to support patients in accepting even modest weight losses they are able to achieve. Most obese individuals lose only about one-third of the weight they would like to lose, which may lead to disappointment and abandonment of continued weight loss efforts. Acceptance of modest weight losses could be facilitated by improving patients' satisfaction with their body image.

Problem-Solving

Training in problem-solving skills provides patients a systematic method to handle with difficulties they discover by self-monitoring. As applied to weight control, patients are taught to: (a) identify and clearly define the weight related difficulty; (b) generate possible solutions for the problem; (c) evaluate the possible solutions and select one; (d) plan and implement the new behavior; (e) evaluate the outcome and, if the intervention was not successful, reevaluate the problem and select another solution. These techniques are described for example in Fliegel et al. [8].

Control of the Act of Eating

A variety of techniques has been developed to help patients decrease their speed of eating and gain control over it in order to improve satiety and thus be satisfied with less food. These methods include putting fork down between mouthfuls, chewing thoroughly before swallowing, preparing one portion of food at a time, leaving some food on the plate, pausing in the middle of the meal, doing nothing else while eating. Empirically it has been shown that subjects in a behavioral weight loss program who slowed their rate of eating lost significantly more weight than subjects who failed to slow their rate of intake [9].

Additional benefits of slowing eating rate may include increased enjoyment of the flavor and texture of food and greater feelings of self-control.

Nutrition Education

Early behavioral treatment provided minimal dietary counselling. Current behavioral interventions, however, stress the importance of a well-balanced, low-fat diet. The change has made because of findings that the body uses approximately 25% more energy to metabolize carbohydrate than fat. Thus, a person will gain more weight eating fat than in consuming the same number of calories as carbohydrate. The most effective diet results in a gradual change to foods that the patient can continue to eat indefinitely. This means increasing the intake of complex carbohydrates, particularly fruits, vegetables and cereals, and decreasing the intake of fats and concentrated carbohydrates (see [10] for further description).

Physical Activity

Increased physical activity is perhaps the single best correlate of long-term weight control. Therefore an exercise component is incorporated in every behavioral weight loss program. A first step is to help patients to monitor their physical activity. Mechanical pedometers are an inexpensive way of making such measurements. Once the level of physical activity is being monitored behavioral interventions are used to increase the level. A key element is to begin slowly so that patients do not repeat their frequent experience of failure. For this reason programmed activities and sports are not the first choice. Instead 'lifestyle' activities are encouraged: getting off the bus a stop too early or a stop too late, parking the car some distance from one's destination, using the stairs instead of the elevators. To sum up, any means of 'wasting' energy that appeals to the patient [11].

Short-Term Results of Behavioral Treatment

A meta-analysis using data from randomized controlled trials published from 1974 to 2002 [12] indicates a very favorable outcome. Patients treated by a comprehensive behavioral approach lost approximately 10.7 kg (~10% of initial weight). In addition, the completion rate for the treatment was 80%. A comparison of former (1974) with more recent studies (1996–2002) reveals that weight losses in behavioral treatments have more than doubled in the past 25 years.

Long-Term Results of Behavioral Treatment

Weight regain is a problem following virtually all dietary and behavioral interventions. Patients treated by behavioral therapy for 20–30 weeks typically regain about 30–35% of the lost weight in the year following treatment [13]. Weight regain slows after the first year but by 5 years, 50% of patients are likely to have returned to their baseline weight.

Several studies have demonstrated the benefits of patients continuing to attend weight maintenance classes after completing an initial weight loss program. Perri et al. [13], for example, found that individuals who attended every other week group maintenance sessions for the year following weight reduction maintained 13.0 kg of their 13.2 kg end of treatment weight loss, whereas those who did not receive such follow-up treatment maintained only 5.7 kg of a 10.8-kg loss. Maintenance sessions should provide patients the support and motivation needed to continue and practice weight control skills, such as keeping food records and exercising regularly. In these sessions, it should be focused on identification of high-risk situations, on training to avoid lapses, and on positive coping with slips and relapses. Further content of maintenance sessions are methods to increase social and emotional support for weight maintenance by partners or friends. A third focus should be to strengthen the motivation to adhere to physical activity and lifestyle changes.

When reviewing 13 studies on this topic, Perri and Corsica [14] found that patients who received long-term treatment, which averages 41 sessions over 54 weeks maintained 10.3 kg of their initial 10.7-kg weight loss.

However, a clear limitation of long-term behavioral treatment seems to be that it only delays rather than prevents weight regain [12]. Behavioral maintenance therapy is generally successful in sustaining losses of about 10–12% of initial weight but not reductions of 20% or more. Even with very intensive programmes, larger losses are difficult to maintain, in part, because of compensatory biological responses to weight reduction (e.g. decreases in leptin and resting energy expenditure [15, 16]).

Resume and Outlook

Behavioral treatment of obesity is clearly effective in inducing a loss of 8–10% of initial weight. Losses of this size are associated with significant improvements in health. Further research in particular should address how to improve the long-term efficacy of behavioral treatment packages as a whole and the question which treatment components are most successful.

Resources and efforts also must be devoted to the prevention of obesity, using behaviorally oriented means. The best hope for prevention may lie with children and adolescents. Special efforts should be made to improve meals and snacks served at schools, to provide more opportunities for physical activity at school and at home, and educate youth about the importance of diet, activity, and healthy body weight. Ultimately, we should try to change an environment that encourages people to consume high-fat, high-sugar foods in super-sized servings.

Although behavioral treatment can assist those who already are obese, there is more need for wide scale environmental interventions that will reduce the number of individuals who will require such treatment.

References

1 Stuart RB: Behavioral control of overeating. Behav Res Ther 1967;5:357–365.
2 Kanfer FH, Goldstein, AP: Helping People Change. New York, Pergamon, 1975.
3 Wadden TA, Foster GD: Behavioral Assessment and treatment of markedly obese patients; in Wadden TA, VanItallie TB (eds): Treatment of the Seriously Obese Patient. New York, Guilford Press, 1992, pp 290–330.
4 Brownell KD, Wadden TA: Etiology and treatment of obesity: Understanding a serious, prevalent, and refractory disorder. J Consult Clin Psychol 1992;60:505–517.
5 Foster GD, Wadden TA, Vogt RA: What is a reasonable weight loss? Patients' expectations and evaluations of obesity treatment outcomes. J Consult Clin Psychol 1997;65:79–85.
6 Wadden TA: Characteristics of successful weight loss maintainers; in Allison DB, Pi-Sunyer FX (eds): Obesity Treatment: Establishing Goals, Improving Outcomes, and Reviewing the Research Agenda. New York, Plenum Press, 1995, pp 103–111.
7 Cooper Z, Fairburn CG, Hawker DM: Cognitive-Behavioral Treatment of Obesity. New York, Guilford Press, 2003.
8 Fliegel S, Groeger WM, Kuenzel R, Schulte D, Sorgatz H: Standard Methods of Behavior Therapy. An Exercise Book. Munich, Urban & Schwarzenberg, 1981.
9 Spiegel TA, Wadden TA, Foster GD: Objective measurement of eating rate during behavioral treatment of obesity. Behav Ther 1991;22:61–67.
10 Pudel V: Adipositas. Göttingen, Hogrefe, 2003.
11 Stunkard A: Behaviour therapy for obesity; in Bender A, Brookes L (eds): Body Weight Control. New York, Churchill-Livingstone, 1987, pp 127–139.
12 Wadden TA, Butryn ML: Behavioral treatment of obesity. Endocrinol Metab Clins N Am 2003; 32:981–1003.
13 Perri MG, McAllister DA, Gange JJ, Jordan RC, McAdoo G, Nezu AM: Effects of four maintenance programs on the long-term management of obesity. J Consult Clin Psychol 1988;56:529–534.
14 Perri MG, Corsica JA: Improving the maintenance of weight lost in behavioral treatment of obesity; in Wadden TA, Stunkard AJ (eds): Handbook of Obesity Treatment. New York, Guilford Press, 2002, pp 357–379.
15 Boden G, Chen X, Mozzoli M, Ryan I: Effects of fasting on serum leptin in normal human subjects. J Clin Endocrinol Metab 1996;81:3419–3423.
16 Wurmser H, Laessle RG, Jacob K, Mueller A, Pirke KM: Resting metabolic rate in preadolescent girls at high risk of obesity. Int J Obesity 1998;22:793–799.

Prof. Dr. Reinhold G. Laessle
University of Trier, Research Department
Clinical Psychology of Nutrition, Universitätsring 15, DE–54286 Trier (Germany)
Tel. +49 651 201 2009, Fax +49 651 201 2886, E-Mail laessle@uni-trier.de

Munsch S, Beglinger C (eds): Obesity and Binge Eating Disorder.
Bibl Psychiatr. Basel, Karger, 2005, No 171, pp 81–101

....

Pharmacological Management of Obesity

George A. Bray

Pennington Biomedical Research Center, Louisiana State University,
Baton Rouge, La., USA

Many physicians and laymen are leery of using medications to manage obesity. This concern stems from several problems associated with their use. First, almost every drug that has been used to treat obesity has been associated with undesirable outcomes that have resulted injury, death and withdrawal of the drug [1]. One of the most serious was the appearance of cardiac valvulopathy following treatment of fenfluramine and phentermine [2–6]. Fenfluramine and dexfenfluramine were subsequently withdrawn from the market. Second, some medications, particularly amphetamine and methamphetamine are addictive, and this has tarnished many drugs with similar chemical structures, whether or not they are demonstrated to be addictive [7]. For example, abuse of either phentermine or diethylpropion is rare [1]. Fenfluramine, a drug with a structure similar to amphetamine has not been reported to be addictive. Third, weight loss during treatment with drugs reaches a plateau after about 6 months, leading many people to conclude erroneously that the drugs have lost their 'effectiveness', even though weight is rapidly regained when the drugs are discontinued [8–15]. Cure for obesity is rare, and treatment is thus aimed at palliation. As clinicians, we do not expect to cure such diseases as hypertension or hypercholesterolemia with medications. Rather, we expect to palliate them. When the medications for any of these diseases are discontinued, we expect the disease to recur. This means that medications only work when used. The same arguments go for medications used to treat overweight. It is a chronic, incurable disease for which drugs only work when used.

In weighing the options regarding treatments for obesity, physicians must be cognizant of these barriers to success. Since binge eating is a problem of overeating often followed by purging, it becomes important to ask whether the medications described below have been used and whether they could be involved in the problem. It is against these limitations that we will review currently available medications. Table 1 summarizes the effects of a number of drugs that are currently available in the United States to treat obesity [1, 16]. They fall into two broad groups, those that produce weight loss by blocking the digestion of fat, and those that act as sympathomimetic appetite suppressants. First I will review the actions and safety of these drugs, and then review some of the agents on both the close and distant horizon, some of which may also be of value in treating binge eating disorders.

Orlistat – A Drug That Blocks Intestinal Digestion

Pharmacology
Orlistat is a potent selective inhibitor of pancreatic lipase that reduces intestinal digestion of fat. The drug has a dose-dependent effect on fecal fat loss, increasing it to about 30% of ingested fat on a diet that has 30% of energy as fat [17]. Orlistat has little effect in subjects eating a low-fat diet, as might be anticipated from the mechanism by which this drug works [17].

Efficacy
A number of long-term clinical trials with orlistat lasting six months to two years have been published [10, 17–27]. In all of the 2-year trials [20] patients received a hypocaloric diet calculated to be 500 kcal/day below the patient's requirements. During the second year the diet was calculated to maintain weight. By the end of year 1, the placebo-treated patients lost between 4 and 6% of their initial body weight and the drug-treated patients lost 8 and 10%. In one study, the patients were re-randomized at the end of year 1. Those switched from orlistat to placebo gained weight from −10 to −6.0% below baseline. Those switched from placebo to orlistat lost from −6 to −8.1%, which was essentially identical to the −7.9% in the patients treated with orlistat for the full 2 years. In a second 2-year study, 892 patients were randomized [21]. One group remained on placebo throughout the 2 years (n = 97 completers) and a second group remained on orlistat 120 mg three times a day for 2 years (n = 109 completers). At the end of 1 year, 2/3 of the group treated with orlistat for 1 year were changed to orlistat 60 mg three times a day (n = 102 completers) and the others to placebo (n = 95 completers) [21]. After 1 year, the weight loss was −8.67 kg in the orlistat-treated group and −5.81 kg in the placebo group (p < 0.001). During the second year, those switched to placebo after one year reached the same weight as those treated with placebo for two years (−4.5% in those with placebo for two years and −4.2% in those switched from orlistat to

Table 1. Drugs approved by the FDA to treat obesity

Drug name	Trade name(s)	Dosage	DEA schedule	Cost/day USD	Side effects and comments
Pancreatic lipase inhibitor					
Orlistat	Xenical	120 mg t.i.d. before meals	none	3.56/day	daily Vitamin pill in the evening; may interact with cyclosporine
Norepinephrine-serotonin reuptake inhibitor					
Sibutramine	Meredia (US) Reductil (rest of world)	5–15 mg/day	IV	2.98–3.56/day	raises blood pressure slightly do not use with monoamine oxidase inhibitors; SSRIs sumatriptan, dihydroergotamine, merpidine; methadon; pentazocine; fentanyl; lithium; tryptophan
Sympathomimetic drugs					
Diethylpropion	Tenuate Tepanil Tenuate Dospan	25 mg t.i.d. 25 mg t.i.d. 75 mg in AM	IV	1.27–1.52/day	all sympathomimetic drugs are similar; do not use with monoamine oxidase inhibitors, guanethidine, alcohol, sibutramine, or tricyclic antidepressants
Phentermine	Standard release Adipex-P Fastin Obenix Oby-Cap	18.75 to 37.5 mg/day, t.i.d.	IV	0.67–1.60/day	see above

Table 1 (continued)

Drug name	Trade name(s)	Dosage	DEA schedule	Cost/day USD	Side effects and comments
	Oby-Trim Zantryl				
	Slow release Ionamin	15–30 mg/day in AM		1.75–2.01/day	
Benzphetamine	Didrex	25–50 mg 1–3 times/day	III	1.19– 2.38/day	see above
Phendimetrazine	Standard release Bontril PDM Plegine X-Trozine	35 mg t.i.d. before meals	III	1.20–5.25/day	see above
	Slow release Bontril Prelu-2 X-Trozine	105 mg/day in AM			

SSRI = Selective serotonin reuptake inhibitor.

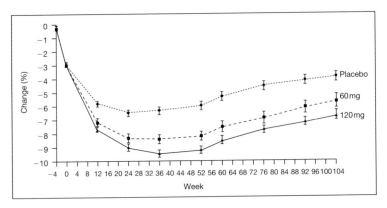

Fig. 1. Hoffmann-La Roche pooled data [17]. The percent change in body weight over 2 years of orlistat at 60 and 120 mg. At the end of 2 years, the orlistat group receiving 120 mg three times daily were 5.2 kg below their baseline weight compared to −1.5 kg for the group treated with placebo.

placebo during year 2). In a third 2-year study, 783 patients enrolled in a trial where, for 2 years, they remained in the placebo group or one of two orlistat-treated groups at 60 or 120 mg three times a day [23]. After one year with a weight loss diet, the completers in the placebo group lost −7.0 kg, which was significantly less than the −9.6 kg in the completers treated with orlistat 60 mg thrice daily or −9.8 kg in the completers treated with orlistat 120 mg thrice daily. During the second year when the diet was liberalized to a 'weight main-tenance' diet, all three groups regained some weight. At the end of 2 years, the completers in the placebo group were −4.3 kg below baseline, the completers treated with orlistat 60 mg three times daily was −6.8 kg and the completers treated with orlistat 120 mg three times daily were −7.6 kg below baseline. Another 2-year trial that has been published was carried out on 796 subjects in a general practice setting [17]. After 1 year of treatment with orlistat 120 mg/day, completers (n = 117) had lost −8.8 kg compared to −4.3 kg in the placebo completers (n = 91). During the second year when the diet was liberalized to 'maintain body weight,' both groups regained some weight. At the end of 2 years, the orlistat group receiving 120 mg three times daily were 5.2 kg below their baseline weight compared to −1.5 kg for the group treated with placebo (fig. 1).

Weight maintenance with orlistat was evaluated in a 1-year study [22]. Patients were enrolled who lost more than 8% of their body weight over six months eating a 1,000-kcal/day (4,180 kJ/day) diet. The 729 patients were one of four groups randomized to receive either placebo or 30, 60 or 120 mg of orli-stat three times a day for 12 months. At the end of this time the placebo-treated patients had regained 56% of their body weight, compared to 32.4% in the group treated with orlistat, 120 mg three times a day. The other two doses of orlistat were not statistically different from placebo in preventing the regain of weight.

Effects of Orlistat on Lipids, Lipoproteins, Glucose Tolerance and Diabetes

The modest weight reduction observed with orlistat treatment may have a beneficial effect on lipids and lipoproteins [28]. From a meta-analysis [29] of the data relating orlistat to lipids, orlistat-treated subjects had almost twice as much reduction in LDL cholesterol as their placebo-treated counterparts for the same weight loss category reached after one year.

A meta-analysis and the Xenical in Diabetes (XENDOS) study have shown that Xenical lowers hemoglobin A1c and reduces the conversion from impaired glucose tolerance to diabetes [30, 31]. In orlistat-treated subjects the conversion from normal glucose tolerance to diabetes occurred in 6.6% of patients, whereas approximately 11% of placebo-treated patients had a similar worsening of glucose tolerance. Conversion from IGT to diabetes was less frequent in orlistat-treated patients than in placebo-treated obese subjects, by 3.0 and 7.6%, respectively [30]. Although these data are based on a retrospective analysis of 1-year trials in which data on glucose tolerance was available, it shows that modest weight reduction – with pharmacotherapy – may lead to an important risk reduction for the development of type II diabetes. In diabetic patients treated with orlistat [26], weight loss in the orlistat-treated group was $-3.9 \pm 0.3\%$ compared to $-1.3 \pm -0.3\%$ in the placebo-treated group, HbA_{1C} was reduced -0.62% in the orlistat-treated group, but only -0.27% in the placebo group. In a 4-year randomized, placebo-controlled clinical trial with orlistat, 1,640 patients were assigned to received orlistat 120 mg three times daily plus lifestyle and 1,637 patients to receive matching placebos plus lifestyle. The study enrolled Swedish patients with a BMI $\geq$30 with normal or impaired glucose tolerance (21%). More than 52% of the orlistat and 34% of the placebo-treated patients continued to adhere to the clinical protocol. The patients receiving orlistat were -6.9 kg below their baseline weight by the end of year 4 compared to -4.1 kg for the placebo-treated group (p < 0.001). Cumulative incidence of diabetes was 9.0% in the placebo group and 6.2% in the orlistat group, a 37% reduction in relative risk. Thus it is clear that long-term clinical trials of anti-obesity drugs can be implemented [31].

Safety

Orlistat is not absorbed to any significant degree and its side effects are thus related to the blockade of triglyceride digestion in the intestine [32]. Fecal fat loss and related GI symptoms are common initially, but subside as patients

---

Bray

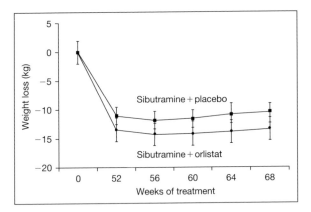

Fig. 2. Addition of orlistat or placebo for 4 months following 1 year of treatment with sibutramine [34]. Patients were randomly assigned to orlistat or placebo in addition to sibutramine following a year of treatment with sibutramine alone. During the additional four months of combination treatment there was no further weight loss.

learn to use the drug [20, 21]. During treatment small but significant decreases in fat-soluble vitamins can occur, although these almost always remain within the normal range [33]. However, a few patients may need supplementation with fat-soluble vitamins that can be lost in the stools. Since it is impossible to tell a priori which patients need vitamins, we routinely provide a multi-vitamin with instructions to take it before bedtime. Absorption of other drugs does not seem to be significantly affected by orlistat.

An analysis of quality of life in patients treated with orlistat showed improvements over the placebo group in spite of the concerns about GI symptoms. In addition, orlistat-treated patients showed a significant decrease in serum cholesterol and LDL cholesterol that is greater than can be explained by the weight loss alone.

Combining Orlistat and Sibutramine

Since orlistat works peripherally to reduce triglyceride digestion in the GI track and sibutramine works on noradrenergic and serotonergic reuptake mechanisms in the brain, their mechanisms don't overlap at all and combining them might provide additive weight loss. To test this possibility, Wadden and his colleagues [34] randomly assigned patients to orlistat or placebo following a year of treatment with orlistat, as depicted in figure 2. During the additional four months of treatment there was no further weight loss. This result was a disappointment, but additional studies are obviously needed before firm conclusions can be made about combining therapies.

Sympathomimetic Drugs That Reduce Food Intake

Pharmacology

The sympathomimetic drugs are grouped together because they can increase blood pressure and, in part, act like NE. Drugs in this group work by a variety of mechanisms including the release of NE from synaptic granules (benzphetamine, phendimetrazine, phentermine, and diethylpropion), the blockade of NE reuptake (mazindol), or blockade of reuptake of both NE and 5-HT (sibutramine). All of these drugs are absorbed orally and reach peak blood concentrations within a short time. The half-life in blood is also short for all except the two pharmacologically active metabolites of sibutramine, which have a long half-life [1]. Although the two metabolites of sibutramine are active, this is not true for the metabolites of other drugs in this group. Liver metabolism inactivates a large fraction of these drugs before excretion. Side effects include dry mouth, constipation, and insomnia. Food intake is suppressed either by delaying the onset of a meal or by producing early satiety. Sibutramine and mazindol have both been shown to increase thermogenesis [28, 35–38].

Efficacy

The first generation of drugs in this class, phentermine, diethylpropion, phenmetrazine and benzphetamine, are only approved for short-term use, and only a few long-term clinical trials have been conducted on the first generation of sympathomimetic drugs [1, 39–45]. The best and one of the longest of these clinical trials lasted 36 weeks and compared placebo treatment against continuous phentermine or intermittent phentermine [12]. Both continuous and intermittent phentermine therapy produced more weight loss than did placebo. In the drug-free periods the patients treated intermittently slowed their weight loss, only to lose more rapidly when the drug was reinstituted. Phentermine is prescribed most frequently in the United States, probably because it is inexpensive, since it is no longer protected by patents. Phentermine is not available in Europe. A recent review in a prestigious journal [46] recommends obtaining written informed consent if phentermine is prescribed for longer than 12 weeks, because this is off-label usage and there are not sufficient published reports on the use of phentermine for long-term use.

Sibutramine is the only second-generation drug that has been approved for long-term treatment of obesity and for maintenance. It has been extensively evaluated in several multi-center trials lasting 6–24 months [9, 47–59]. Several long-term, randomized, placebo-controlled, double-blind clinical trials have been conducted in men and women of all ethnic groups with ages ranging from 18 to 65 years and with a BMI between 27 and 40.

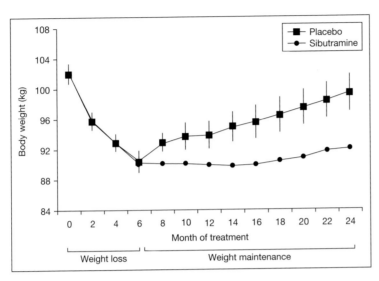

Fig. 3. Sibutramine Trial of Obesity Reduction and Maintenance (STORM) [51]. Patients were initially enrolled in an open-label fashion and treated with 10 mg/day of sibu-tramine for 6 months. Those who lost more than 5% were then randomized 2/3 to sibutramine and 1/3 to placebo. Placebo-treated patients steadily regained weight, maintaining only 20% of their weight loss at the end of the trial, while subjects treated with sibutramine maintained their weight for 12 months and then regained an average of only 2 kg.

A number of conclusions about sibutramine can be drawn from the Sibutramine Trial of Obesity Reduction and Maintenance (STORM Trial) [51], but the effects of sibutramine in aiding weight maintenance are most persuasive (fig. 3). Those patients who lost more than 5% during the first 6 months on sibu-tramine 10 mg/day (77% of enrolled patients met this goal) were randomized 2/3 to sibutramine and 1/3 to placebo. During the 18-month double-blind portion of the trial, the placebo-treated patients steadily regained weight, maintaining only 20% of their weight loss at the end of the trial. In contrast, the subjects treated with sibutramine maintained their weight for 12 months and then regained an average of only 2 kg, thus maintaining 80% of their initial weight loss after two years [51]. In spite of the difference in weight at the end of the 18 months of controlled observation, the mean blood pressure of the sibutramine-treated patients was still higher than in the patients treated with placebo, even though they had a weight difference of several kilograms.

Sibutramine given continuously for one year has been compared to placebo and sibutramine given intermittently [55]. In this study, patients who had lost 2% or 2 kg after four weeks of treatment with sibutramine 15 mg/day were randomized to placebo vs. continuous sibutramine vs. sibutramine prescribed intermittently (weeks 1–12, 19–30 and 37–48). Both sibutramine treatment regimens gave equivalent results and were significantly better than placebo. Stopping sibutramine results in small increases in weight, which is then reversed when the medication is restarted. Four clinical trials with sibutramine in patients with diabetes show a significant reduction in body weight and hemoglobin A1c [55–57, 60].

Two trials have been reported using sibutramine to treat hypertensive patients over one year [9, 59], and two additional studies provide data on 12 weeks of treatment [61, 62]. In all instances, the weight loss pattern favors sibutramine. However, except for one study [62], mean weight loss, though favorable, was associated with mean blood pressure increases. In a three-month trial all patients were receiving β-blockers with or without thiazides for their hypertension [61].

Since the dose of sibutramine influences the amount of weight loss with the drug [47, 48], the intensity of the behavioral component is also likely to have an effect. This is readily demonstrated in a study by Wadden et al. [63]. With minimal behavioral intervention, the weight loss in that study was about 5 kg over 12 months. When group counseling to produce behavior modification was added to sibutramine the weight loss increased to 10 kg, and when a structured meal plan using meal replacements was added to the medication and behavior plan, the weight loss increased further to 15 kg [63]. This indicates that the amount of weight loss observed during pharmacotherapy is due in part to the intensity of the behavioral approach.

Safety

The side effect profile for sympathomimetic drugs is similar [1]. They produce insomnia, dry mouth, asthenia, and constipation. The sympathomimetic drugs phentermine, diethylpropion, benzphetamine and phendimetrazine have very little abuse potential as assessed by the low rate of reinforcement when the drugs are self-injected intravenously to test animals [1]. In this same paradigm, neither phenylpropanolamine nor fenfluramine showed any reinforcing effects and no clinical data show any abuse potential for either of these drugs. Sibutramine, likewise, has no abuse potential [64], but it is nonetheless a scheduled drug by the US Drug Enforcement Agency.

Drugs on the Horizon

Bupropion

Bupropion is a drug approved by the FDA for treatment of depression, which produces weight loss [65]. It is a relative of diethylpropion, an approved drug for treating obesity (see above). It probably acts through modulating

---

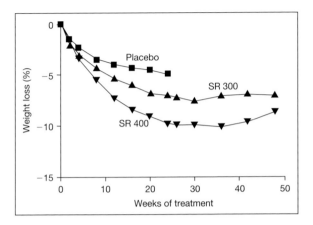

Fig. 4. Bupropion SR percent loss of initial weight [65]. A 6-month randomized, double-blind, placebo-controlled trial with a 6-month blinded extension where all patients received active medication compared two doses of bupropion against placebo (fig. 6). Both doses of medication produced significantly more weight loss than placebo.

the action of norepinephrine [65]. A 6-month randomized, double-blind placebo-controlled trial [65] with a 6-month blinded extension where all patients received active medication has compared two doses of bupropion against placebo (fig. 4). Both doses of medication produced significantly more weight loss than placebo. During the 6-month extension the weight loss was largely maintained. Bupropion has not been given approval by the FDA for weight loss.

Topiramate
Topiramate is a neurotherapeutic agent approved for treatment of epilepsy, both as monotherapy and in combination with other anti-epileptic drugs. Topiramate is a carbonic anhydrase inhibitor that also affects the $GABA_A$ receptor. In uncontrolled clinical studies the drug was noted to cause weight loss [66]. Data from a 6-month placebo-controlled, double-blind randomized dose-ranging clinical trial has been published [67] (fig. 5) and a number of studies from the terminated 2-year trials have been presented in abstract form. In the dose-ranging study, topiramate was titrated to final doses of 64, 96, 192 and 384 mg/day. All 4 doses produced significantly greater weight loss than placebo. The weight loss was similar with the two lower doses and with the two higher doses. Higher doses were associated with an increasing number of neurological side effects. In a 60-week trial, the lower dose of 96 mg/day produced nearly 9% weight loss. Higher doses of 192 and 256 mg/day produced even more weight loss of 12–13% (68). These effects exceed those of any other monotherapy yet reported. In a trial where topiramate was introduced after an

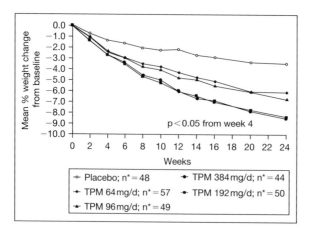

Fig. 5. Weight loss with topiramate [66]. In a placebo-controlled, double-blind, random-ized dose-ranging clinical trial presented in abstract form, topiramate at doses of 64, 96, 192 and 184 mg/day produced dose-related weight loss, but was also associated with dose-related increases in the number of neurological side effects.

8-week period of weight loss on a low-calorie diet that produced an average of 10% weight loss, placebo treatment maintained therapeutic weight loss for 44 weeks, whereas doses of 96 and 192 mg/day of topiramate produced further weight loss of 16 to 18%. Topiramate lowered blood pressure, but not lipids.

Rimonabant

Endocannabinoids may be involved in the leptin pathway, which regulates food intake. Rimonabant is a cannabinoid antagonist binding to CB_{1A} receptors [69]. It has been evaluated in yearlong trials as an anti-obesity drug and as a drug to reduce smoking. Doses of 5 and 20 mg/day were tested in both of trials. During the 52 weeks of treatment, 20 mg/day of rimonabant produced a 9 kg weight loss compared to 4 kg with 5 mg and 2 kg with placebo (fig. 6). The therapeutic effect reached a maximum by 36 weeks and the therapeutic effect was unaltered at 52 weeks. Of those treated with 20 mg/d, 72.9% of those on treatment lost more that 5 and 44.3% lost more than 10% of initial weight at 1 year. HDL-cholesterol increased more than 20% and triglycerides decreased by more than 15% with the higher dose of rimonabant. Glucose and insulin were also reduced and the number of patients with the metabolic syndrome as defined by the Adult Treatment Panel III of the National Cholesterol Education Program fell from 52.9% at baseline to 25.8% at 1 year in patients treated with the 20 mg/day dose of rimonabant. Rimonabant also reduced blood pressure in association with the weight loss. In the anti-smoking study weight gain was 3.0 kg

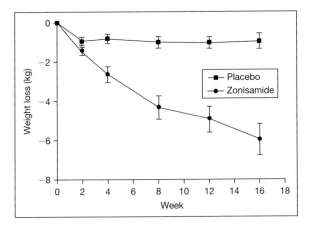

Fig. 6. Effect of zonisamide of weight loss. In this 16-week trial, zonisamide, an anticonvulsant, produced significantly more weight loss than placebo [70].

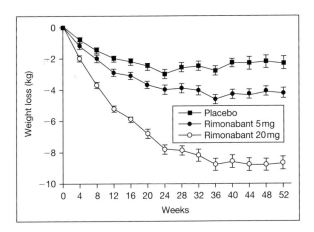

Fig. 7. Effect of rimonabant on weight loss. In this 52-week trial, subjects received placebo, or one of 2 doses of rimonabant. Weight loss had plateaued by 36 weeks [68].

in the placebo group compared to 0.7 kg in those treated with rimonabant 20 mg/day. This reduced weight gain was associated with a 36.2% abstinence rate compared with a 20.6% abstinence rate in the placebo group during the last 4 weeks of the 10-week treatment period.

Zonisamide
Zonisamide is a neurotherapeutic drug that is approved by the Food and Drug Administration as treatment for epilepsy. One 16-week randomized,

placebo-controlled clinical trial has been reported with this drug. Weight loss was significantly greater than in the placebo treated group [70] (fig. 7).

Leptin

Leptin is a peptide produced almost exclusively in adipose tissue. Absence of leptin produces massive obesity in mice (ob/ob) and in humans [71], and treatment with this peptide decreases food intake in the ob/ob mouse and the leptin-deficient human [72]. The diabetes mouse (db/db) and the fatty rat, which have genetic defects in the leptin receptor, are also obese but they do not respond to leptin. Leptin levels in the blood are highly correlated with body fat levels yet obesity persists, suggesting that there may be leptin resistance. A dose-ranging clinical trial with leptin has been reported [73]. In lean subjects treated for four weeks and in obese subjects treated for 24 weeks there was a modest loss of weight with doses ranging from 0.01 to 0.3 mg/kg. The side effects of local irritation at the site of injection limit the use of this preparation. A long-acting leptin preparation may provide an improved way to use this drug [74].

Axokine

Axokine is a modified form of ciliary neurotrophic factor (CNTF). It acts through the same janus-kinase signal for transduction and translation (JAK-STAT) system that leptin acts through. CNTF will reduce food intake in animals that lack leptin or the leptin receptors [75]. In a clinical trial for amyotrophic lateral sclerosis, the drug was noted to reduce weight and a 3-month dose-ranging study was conducted that demonstrated a significantly greater dose-related weight loss in the drug-treated patients. In a dose-ranging clinical trial CNTF produced a significant therapeutic response with weight loss of 3–5%. Following termination of the drug, weight loss appeared to be maintained better in the patients who got CNTF than in the placebo-treated group. The first half of a 2-year randomized placebo-controlled trial was reported in April 2003. About 70% of the CNTF treated patients developed antibodies to the drug. Weight loss of about 5% occurred prior to the development of antibodies, but once antibodies appeared the drug appeared to lose its effectiveness on body weight.

Neuropeptide-Y

Neuropeptide-Y (NPY) is one of the most potent stimulators of food intake and appears to act through NPY Y-5 and/or Y-1 receptors [1]. Antagonists to these receptors might block NPY and thus decrease feeding. Several pharmaceutical companies are attempting to identify antagonists to NPY receptors [16].

Melanin Concentrating Hormone

Melanin concentrating hormone is found primarily in the lateral hypothalamic areas of the brain. When injected into the brain, it increases food intake.

In transgenic mice that do not express MCH, there is modest weight loss. Conversely, when mice overexpress this peptide, they become fatter. Thus, antagonists to this peptide provide interesting potential agents for future evaluation [76].

Cholecystokinin

Cholecystokinin (CCK) reduces food intake in human beings and in experimental animals [1]. This effect does not require an intact hypothalamic feeding control system but does appear to require an intact vagus nerve. Peptide analogs have been developed and tested experimentally but clinical data have not yet been published. A second strategy to modify CCK activity is to reduce the degradation of CCK. This approach is likewise under evaluation.

Glucagon and Glucagon-Like Peptide-1 (GLP-1)

Pancreatic glucagon produces a dose-related decrease in food intake [1]. A fragment of glucagon (amino acids 6–29) called glucagon-like peptide-1 (GLP-1) reduced food intake when given either peripherally [77] or into the brain. Exendin, an analog of GLP-1, has been used in humans since infusion of GLP-1 in humans reduces food intake [78].

Pramlintide

Pramlintide, an analog of amylin, is in clinical trial for diabetes. There is modest weight loss in these clinical trials and more are planned.

Melanocortin Receptors

Mice whose melanocortin-4 receptor has been genetically disabled become markedly obese. In one clinical trial, subjects took intranasal doses of MSH/ACHT$_{4-10}$ twice daily for 6 weeks. Placebo treatment produced no changes in body fat, but those received MSH/ACHT$_{4-10}$ lost 1.68 kg body fat ($p < 0.05$) and 0.79 kg body weight ($p < 0.001$) [79]. These findings suggest that MC-4 receptor agonists might be useful in treatment obesity.

Ephedrine and Caffeine
Pharmacology

Ephedrine is a derivative of phenylpropanolamine and is used to relax bronchial smooth muscles in patients with asthma. It also stimulates thermogenesis in human subjects [80, 81]. Caffeine is a xanthine that inhibits adenosine receptors and phosphodiesterase. In experimental animals the combination of ephedrine and caffeine reduces body weight, probably through stimulation of thermogenesis and a reduction in food intake [1].

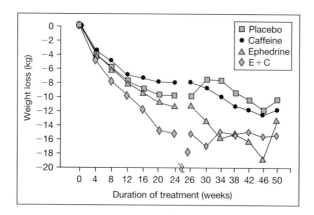

Fig. 8. Effect of ephedrine and caffeine on weight loss and weight maintenance for 1 year [14]. A total of 180 patients were randomly assigned to 4 groups that were then treated in a double-blind fashion for 6 months and with an open-label protocol for another 6 months. The weight losses in the groups receiving placebo, ephedrine alone, and caffeine alone were not significantly different and were smaller than in the group receiving the combination of ephedrine and caffeine. During the 6-month open-label study when those who wished to received ephedrine and caffeine, weight loss was maintained with no significant difference between groups.

Efficacy

One long-term placebo-controlled clinical trial enrolled 180 patients treated with ephedrine, caffeine, or the combination of ephedrine and caffeine [82]. Patients treated with the combination of ephedrine and caffeine lost more weight than did patients treated with ephedrine alone, caffeine alone or placebo (fig. 8). In a six-month open-label extension, subjects who completed the initial trial were offered additional treatment with ephedrine and caffeine. Nearly two-thirds of the group opted for this treatment and were able to maintain their initial weight loss for the next six months. No other long-term data are available using ephedrine and caffeine. During controlled metabolic studies, patients treated with ephedrine and caffeine lost less lean tissue than did those in the placebo-treated group. Using the changes in body composition from these studies, Astrup et al. [81] have estimated the contribution of thermogenesis and food intake to the weight loss. They concluded that 60–75% of the weight loss was due to a decrease in food intake and 25–40% was due to the thermogenic effects of ephedrine and caffeine.

Safety

Although caffeine and ephedrine have a long record of clinical use separately, neither drug alone nor the combination is approved for treatment of obesity.

The US Food and Drug Administration has withdrawn herbal preparations containing ephedra (a herbal form of ephedrine) from the market because of concerns about increased risks to health.

Conclusion

At present only two drugs are approved for long-term treatment of obesity. Sibutramine inhibits the re-uptake of serotonin and norepinephrine. In clinical trials it produces a dose-dependent 5–10% decrease in body weight. Its side effects include the dry mouth, insomnia, asthenia, and constipation. In addition, in clinical trials, sibutramine produces a small mean increase in blood pressure and pulse that mandates attention to blood pressure monitoring on follow-up visits. Sibutramine is contraindicated in some individuals with heart disease. Orlistat is the other drug approved for long-term use in the treatment of obesity. It works by blocking pancreatic lipase and thus increasing the fecal loss of triglyceride. One valuable consequence of this mechanism of action is the reduction of serum cholesterol that averages about 5% more than can be accounted for by weight loss alone. In clinical trials it produces a 5–10% loss of weight. Its side effects are entirely due to undigested fat in the intestine (steatorrhea) that can lead to increased frequency and change in the character of stools. It can also lower fat-soluble vitamins. The ingestion of a vitamin supplement before bedtime is a reasonable treatment strategy when orlistat is prescribed. All medications currently available for obesity management should be used as adjuncts to dietary and physical activity approaches to weight management. Patients who meet prescribing guidelines (BMI $\geq$30 or $\geq$27 with a cormorbid condition) and who are motivated to undertake concurrent lifestyle change may receive health benefits from the additional weight loss that accompanies medication use.

References

1   Bray GA, Greenway FL: Current and potential drugs for treatment of obesity. Endocr Rev 1999;20:805–875.
2   Connolly HM, Crary JL, McGoon MD, Hensrud DD, Edwards BS, Schaff HV: Valvular heart disease associated with fenfluramine-phentermine. N Engl J Med 1997;337:581–588.
3   Ryan DH, Bray GA, Helmcke F, Sander G, Volaufova J, Greenway F, Subramaniam P, Glancy DL: Serial echocardiographic and clinical evaluation of valvular regurgitation before, during, and after treatment with fenfluramine or dexfenfluramine and mazindol or phentermine. Obes Res 1999;7:313–322.
4   Jick H: Heart valve disorders and appetite-suppressant drugs. JAMA 2000;283:1738–1740.
5   Hensrud DD, Connolly HM, Grogan M, Miller FA, Bailey KR, Jensen MD: Echocardiographic improvement over time after cessation of use of fenfluramine and phentermine. Mayo Clin Proc 1999;74:1191–1197.

6   Mast ST, Jollis JG, Ryan T, Anstrom KJ, Crary JL: The progression of fenfluramine-associated valvular heart disease assessed by echocardiography. Ann Intern Med 2001;134:261–256.

7   Weintraub M, Bray GA: Drug treatment of obesity. Med Clins N Am 1989;73:237–249.

8   Bray GA: Obesity: A time bomb to be defused. Lancet 1998;352:160–161.

9   McMahon FG, Fujioka K, Singh BN, Mendel CM, Rowe E, Rolston K, Johnson F, Mooradian AD: Efficacy and safety of sibutramine in obese white and African American patients with hypertension: A 1-year, double-blind, placebo-controlled, multicenter trial. Arch Intern Med 2000;160:2185–2191.

10   Finer N, James WP, Kopelman PG, Lean ME, Williams G: One-year treatment of obesity: A randomized, double-blind, placebo-controlled, multicentre study of orlistat, a gastrointestinal lipase inhibitor. Int J Obes Relat Metab Disord 2000;24:306–313.

11   Flechtner-Mors M, Ditschuneit HH, Johnson TD, Suchard MA, Adler G: Metabolic and weight loss effects of long-term dietary intervention in obese patients: Four-year results. Obes Res 2000; 8:399–402.

12   Munro J, MacCuish A, Wilson E, Duncan L: Comparison of continuous and intermittent anorectic therapy in obesity. Br Med J 1968;1:352–354.

13   Greenway FL, Ryan DH, Bray GA, Rood JC, Tucker EW, Smith SR: Pharmaceutical cost savings of treating obesity with weight loss medications. Obes Res 1999;7:523–531.

14   Astrup A, Breum L, Toubro S, Hein P, Quaade F: The effect and safety of an ephedrine/caffeine compound compared to ephedrine, caffeine and placebo in obese subjects on an energy restricted diet: A double blind trial. Int J Obes Relat Metab Disord 1992;16:269–277.

15   Sjostrom CD, Lissner L, Wedel H, Sjostrom L: Reduction in incidence of diabetes, hypertension and lipid disturbances after intentional weight loss induced by bariatric surgery: The SOS Intervention Study. Obes Res 1999;7:477–484.

16   Bray GA, Tartaglia LA: Medicinal strategies in the treatment of obesity. Nature 2000;404:672–677.

17   Hauptman J, Lucas C, Boldrin MN, Collins H, Segal KR: Orlistat in the long-term treatment of obesity in primary care settings. Arch Fam Med 2000;9:160–167.

18   James WP, Avenell A, Broom J, Whitehead J: A one-year trial to assess the value of orlistat in the management of obesity. Int J Obes Relat Metab Disord 1997;21(suppl 3):S24–S30.

19   Van Gaal LF, Broom JI, Enzi G, Toplak H: Efficacy and tolerability of orlistat in the treatment of obesity: A 6-month dose-ranging study. Orlistat Dose-Ranging Study Group. Eur J Clin Pharmacol 1998;54:125–132.

20   Sjostrom L, Rissanen A, Andersen T, Boldrin M, Golay A, Koppeschaar HP, Krempf M: Randomised placebo-controlled trial of orlistat for weight loss and prevention of weight regain in obese patients. European Multicentre Orlistat Study Group. Lancet 1998;352:167–172.

21   Davidson MH, Hauptman J, DiGirolamo M, Foreyt JP, Halsted CH, Heber D, Heimburger DC, Lucas CP, Robbins DC, Chung J, Heymsfield SB: Weight control and risk factor reduction in obese subjects treated for 2 years with orlistat: A randomized controlled trial. JAMA 1999;281:235–242.

22   Hill JO, Hauptman J, Anderson JW, Fujioka K, O'Neil PM, Smith DK, Zavoral JH, Aronne LJ: Orlistat, a lipase inhibitor, for weight maintenance after conventional dieting: A 1-y study. Am J Clin Nutr 1999;69:1108–1116.

23   Rossner S, Sjostrom L, Noack R, Meinders AE, Noseda G: Weight loss, weight maintenance, and improved cardiovascular risk factors after 2 years treatment with orlistat for obesity. European Orlistat Obesity Study Group. Obes Res 2000;8:49–61.

24   Lindgarde F: The effect of orlistat on body weight and coronary heart disease risk profile in obese patients: The Swedish Multimorbidity Study. J Intern Med 2000;248:245–254.

25   Hollander PA, Elbein SC, Hirsch IB, Kelley D, McGill J, Taylor T, Weiss SR, Crockett SE, Kaplan RA, Comstock J, Lucas CP, Lodewick PA, Canovachtel W, Chung J, Hauptman J: Role of orlistat in the treatment of obese patients with type 2 diabetes: A 1-year randomized double-blind study. Diabetes Care 1998;21:1288–1294.

26   Kelley DE, Bray GA, Pi-Sunyer FX, Klein S, Hill J, Miles J, Hollander P: Clinical efficacy of orlistat therapy in overweight and obese patients with insulin-treated type 2 diabetes: A 1-year randomized controlled trial. Diabetes Care 2002;25:1033–1041.

27   Miles JM, Leiter L, Hollander P, Wadden T, Anderson JW, Doyle M, Foreyt J, Aronne L, Klein S: Effect of orlistat in overweight and obese patients with type 2 diabetes treated with metformin. Diabetes Care 2002;25:1123–1128.

28 Astrup A, Hansen DL, Lundsgaard C, Toubro S: Sibutramine and energy balance. Int J Obes Relat Metab Disord 1998;22 (suppl 1):S30–S35; discussion S36–S37, S42.

29 Zavoral JH: Treatment with orlistat reduces cardiovascular risk in obese patients. J Hypertens 1998;16:2013–2017.

30 Heymsfield SB, Segal KR, Hauptman J, Lucas CP, Boldrin MN, Rissanen A, Wilding JP, Sjostrom L: Effects of weight loss with orlistat on glucose tolerance and progression to type 2 diabetes in obese adults. Arch Intern Med 2000;160:1321–1326.

31 Torgerson JS, Hauptman J, Boldrin MN, Sjostrom L: XENical in the prevention of diabetes in obese subjects (XENDOS) study: A randomized study of orlistat as an adjunct to lifestyle changes for the prevention of type 2 diabetes in obese patients. Diabetes Care 2004;27:155–161.

32 Hauptman J: Orlistat: Selective inhibition of caloric absorption can affect long-term body weight. Endocrine 2000;13:201–206.

33 Drent ML, van der Veen EA: First clinical studies with orlistat: A short review. Obes Res 1995; 3(suppl 4):623S–625S.

34 Wadden TA, Berkowitz RI, Womble LG, Sarwer DB, Arnold ME, Steinberg CM: Effects of sibutramine plus orlistat in obese women following 1 year of treatment by sibutramine alone: A placebo-controlled trial. Obes Res 2000;8:431–437.

35 National Task Force on the Prevention and Treatment of Obesity: Long-term pharmacotherapy in the management of obesity. JAMA 1996;276:1907–1915.

36 Hansen DL, Toubro S, Stock MJ, Macdonald IA, Astrup A: Thermogenic effects of sibutramine in humans. Am J Clin Nutr 1998;68:1180–1186.

37 Lang SS, Danforth E Jr, Lien EL: Anorectic drugs which stimulate thermogenesis. Life Sci 1983;33:1269–1275.

38 Lupien JR, Bray GA: Effect of mazindol, d-amphetamine and diethylpropion on purine nucleotide binding to brown adipose tissue. Pharmacol Biochem Behav 1986;25:733–738.

39 Bray GA: Evaluation of drugs for treating obesity. Obes Res 1995;3(suppl 4):425S–434S.

40 Silverstone J, Solomon T: The long-term management of obesity in general practice. J Clin Pract 1965;19:395–398.

41 McKay RH: Long-term use of diethylpropion in obesity. Curr Med Res Opin 1973;1:489–493.

42 Langlois KJ, Forbes JA, Bell GW, Grant GF Jr: A double-blind clinical evaluation of the safety and efficacy of phentermine hydrochloride (Fastin) in the treatment of exogenous obesity. Curr Ther Res Clin Exp 1974;16:289–296.

43 Gershberg H, Kane R, Hulse M, Pensgen E: Effects of diet and an anorectic drug (phentermine resin) in obese diabetics. Curr Ther Res 1977;22:814–820.

44 Campbell CJ, Bhalla IP, Steel JM, Duncan LJ: A controlled trial of phentermine in obese diabetic patients. Practitioner 1977;218:851–855.

45 Williams RA, Foulsham BM: Weight reduction in osteoarthritis using phentermine. Practitioner 1981;225:231–232.

46 Yanovski SZ, Yanovski JA: Obesity. N Engl J Med 2002;346:591–602.

47 Bray GA, Ryan DH, Gordon D, Heidingsfelder S, Cerise F, Wilson K: A double-blind randomized placebo-controlled trial of sibutramine. Obes Res 1996;4:263–270.

48 Bray GA, Blackburn GL, Ferguson JM, Greenway FL, Jain AK, Mendel CM, Mendels J, Ryan DH, Schwartz SL, Scheinbaum ML, Seaton TB: Sibutramine produces dose-related weight loss. Obes Res 1999;7:189–198.

49 Apfelbaum M, Vague P, Ziegler O, Hanotin C, Thomas F, Leutenegger E: Long-term maintenance of weight loss after a very-low-calorie diet: A randomized blinded trial of the efficacy and tolerability of sibutramine. Am J Med 1999;106:179–184.

50 Fanghanel G, Cortinas L, Sanchez-Reyes L, Berber A: A clinical trial of the use of sibutramine for the treatment of patients suffering essential obesity. Int J Obes Relat Metab Disord 2000;24:144–150.

51 James WP, Astrup A, Finer N, Hilsted J, Kopelman P, Rossner S, Saris WH, Van Gaal LF: Effect of sibutramine on weight maintenance after weight loss: A randomised trial. STORM Study Group. Sibutramine Trial of Obesity Reduction and Maintenance. Lancet 2000;356:2119–2125.

52 Cuellar GE, Ruiz AM, Monsalve MC, Berber A: Six-month treatment of obesity with sibutramine 15 mg: A double-blind, placebo-controlled monocenter clinical trial in a Hispanic population. Obes Res 2000;8:71–82.

53   Smith IG, Goulder MA: Randomized placebo-controlled trial of long-term treatment with sibutramine in mild to moderate obesity. J Fam Pract 2001;50:505–512.

54   Dujovne CA, Zavoral JH, Rowe E, Mendel CM: Effects of sibutramine on body weight and serum lipids: A double-blind, randomized, placebo-controlled study in 322 overweight and obese patients with dyslipidemia. Am Heart J 2001;142:489–497.

55   Wirth A, Krause J: Long-term weight loss with sibutramine: A randomized controlled trial. Jama 2001;286:1331–1339.

56   Fujioka K, Seaton TB, Rowe E, Jelinek CA, Raskin P, Lebovitz HE, Weinstein SP, Sibutramine/Diabetes Clinical Study Group: Weight loss with sibutramine improves glycaemic control and other metabolic parameters in obese patients with type 2 diabetes mellitus. Diabetes Obes Metab 2000;2:175–187.

57   Gokcel A, Karakose H, Ertorer EM, Tanaci N, Tutuncu NB, Guvener N: Effects of sibutramine in obese female subjects with type 2 diabetes and poor blood glucose control. Diabetes Care 2001;24:1957–1960.

58   Serrano-Rios M, Melchionda N, Moreno-Carretero E: Role of sibutramine in the treatment of obese Type 2 diabetic patients receiving sulphonylurea therapy. Diabet Med 2002;19:119–124.

59   McMahon FG, Weinstein SP, Rowe E, Ernst KR, Johnson F, Fujioka K: Sibutramine is safe and effective for weight loss in obese patients whose hypertension is well controlled with angiotensin-converting enzyme inhibitors. J Hum Hypertens 2002;16:5–11.

60   Finer N, Bloom SR, Frost GS, Banks LM, Griffiths J: Sibutramine is effective for weight loss and diabetic control in obesity with type 2 diabetes: A randomised, double-blind, placebo-controlled study. Diabetes Obes Metab 2000;2:105–112.

61   Hazenberg BP: Randomized, double-blind, placebo-controlled, multicenter study of sibutramine in obese hypertensive patients. Cardiology 2000;94:152–158.

62   Sramek JJ, Leibowitz MT, Weinstein SP, Rowe ED, Mendel CM, Levy B, McMahon FG, Mullican WS, Toth PD, Cutler NR: Efficacy and safety of sibutramine for weight loss in obese patients with hypertension well controlled by beta-adrenergic blocking agents: A placebo-controlled, double-blind, randomised trial. J Hum Hypertens 2002;16:13–19.

63   Wadden TA, Berkowitz RI, Sarwer DB, Prus-Wisniewski R, Steinberg C: Benefits of lifestyle modification in the pharmacologic treatment of obesity: A randomized trial. Arch Intern Med 2001;161:218–227.

64   Cole JO, Levin A, Beake B, Kaiser PE, Scheinbaum ML: Sibutramine: A new weight loss agent without evidence of the abuse potential associated with amphetamines. J Clin Psychopharmacol 1998;18:231–236.

65   Anderson JW, Greenway FL, Fujioka K, Gadde KM, McKenney J, O'Neil PM: Bupropion SR enhances weight loss: A 48-week double-blind, placebo-controlled trial. Obes Res 2002;10:633–641.

66   Reife R, Pledger G, Wu SC: Topiramate as add-on therapy: Pooled analysis of randomized controlled trials in adults. Epilepsia 2000;41(suppl 1):S66–S71.

67   Bray G, Klein S, Levy B, Fitchet M, Perry BH: Topiramate produces dose-related weight loss in obese patients. Diabetes 2002;51(suppl 2):A420–A421.

68   Wilding J, Van Gaal L, Rissanen A, Vercruysse F, Fitchet M: A randomized double-blind placebo-controlled study of the long-term efficacy and safety of topiramate in the treatment of obese subjects. Intern J Obes 2004;28:1399–1410.

69   Di Marzo V, Goparaju SK, Wang L, Liu J, Batkai S, Jarai Z, Fezza F, Miura GI, Palmiter RD, Sigiura T, Kunos G: Leptin-regulated endocannabinoids are involved in maintaining food intake. Nature 2001;410:822–825.

70   Gadde KM, Francisy DM, Wagner HR 2nd, Krishnan KR: Zonisamide for weight loss in obese adults: A randomized controlled trial. JAMA 2003;289:1820–1825.

71   Montague CT, Farooqi IS, Whitehead JP, Soos MA, Rau H, Wareham NJ, Sewter CP, Digby JE, Mohammed SN, Hurst JA, Cheetham CH, Earley AR, Barnett AH, Prins JB, O'Rahilly S: Congenital leptin deficiency is associated with severe early-onset obesity in humans. Nature 1997;387:903–908.

72   Farooqi IS, Jebb SA, Langmack G, Lawrence E, Cheetham CH, Prentice AM, Hughes IA, McCamish MA, O'Rahilly S: Effects of recombinant leptin therapy in a child with congenital leptin deficiency. N Engl J Med 1999;341:879–884.

73 Heymsfield SB, Greenberg AS, Fujioka K, Dixon RM, Kushner R, Hunt T, Lubina JA, Patane J, Self B, Hunt P, McCamish M: Recombinant leptin for weight loss in obese and lean adults: A randomized, controlled, dose-escalation trial. JAMA 1999;282:1568–1575.

74 Hukshorn CJ, Saris WH, Westerterp-Plantenga MS, Farid AR, Smith FJ, Campfield LA: Weekly subcutaneous pegylated recombinant native human leptin (PEG-OB) administration in obese men. J Clin Endocrinol Metab 2000;85:4003–4009.

75 Lambert PD, Anderson KD, Sleeman MW, Wong V, Tan J, Hijarunguru A, Corcoran TL, Murray JD, Thabet KE, Yancopoulos GD, Wiegand SJ: Ciliary neurotrophic factor activates leptin-like pathways and reduces body fat, without cachexia or rebound weight gain, even in leptin-resistant obesity. Proc Natl Acad Sci USA 2001;98:4652–4657.

76 Ludwig DS, Tritos NA, Mastaitis JW, Kulkami R, Kokkotou E, Elmquist J, Lowell B, Flier JS, Maratos-Flier E: Melanin-concentrating hormone overexpression in transgenic mice leads to obesity and insulin resistance. J Clin Invest 2001;107:379–386.

77 Flint A, Raben A, Astrup A, Holst JJ: Glucagon-like peptide 1 promotes satiety and suppresses energy intake in humans. J Clin Invest 1998;101:515–520.

78 Al-Barazanji KA, Arch JR, Buckingham RE, Tadayyon M: Central exendin-4 infusion reduces body weight without altering plasma leptin in (fa/fa) Zucker rats. Obes Res 2000;8:317–323.

79 Fehm HL, Smolnik R, Kern W, McGregor GP, Bickel U, Born J: The melanocortin melanocyte-stimulating hormone/adrenocorticotropin(4–10) decreases body fat in humans. J Clin Endocrinol Metab 2001;86:1144–1148.

80 Astrup A, Bulow J, Madsen J, Christensen NJ: Contribution of BAT and skeletal muscle to thermogenesis induced by ephedrine in man. Am J Physiol 1985;248:E507–E515.

81 Astrup A, Breum L, Toubro S: Pharmacological and clinical studies of ephedrine and other thermogenic agonists. Obes Res 1995;3(suppl 4):537S–540S.

82 Astrup A, Breum L, Toubro S, Hein P, Quaade F: Ephedrine and weight loss. Int J Obes Relat Metab Disord 1992;16:715.

George A. Bray, MD
Pennington Biomedical Research Center
Louisiana State University, 6400 Perkins Road
Baton Rouge, LA 70808 (USA)
Tel. +1 225 763 3140, Fax +1 225 763 3045, E-Mail brayga@pbrc.edu

Munsch S, Beglinger C (eds): Obesity and Binge Eating Disorder.
Bibl Psychiatr. Basel, Karger, 2005, No 171, pp 102–116

....

Surgical Treatment of Morbid Obesity

Markus K. Müller, Markus Weber

Department of Visceral and Transplantation Surgery (Director: Prof. P.-A. Clavien),
University Hospital Zürich, Zürich, Switzerland

In recent years, obesity surgery (= bariatric surgery, from baros (greek) = weight, heaviness) has emerged from being the interest of only few surgeons to a well-recognized surgical speciality. This development was driven by the increasing prevalence of obesity which has reached epidemic dimensions in Western countries and by the introduction of new techniques, especially laparoscopic surgical procedures. The burden for our societies rising from the harm and cost caused by obesity-associated comorbidities has forced us to find efficient medical treatment. Since conservative treatment strategies have mostly failed in the long term, obesity surgery has become one of the most promising options to treat this threatening social and economic catastrophe. The NIH consensus conference in 1996 concluded that surgical therapy offers the best long-term approach to treat morbid obesity and is probably the most effective therapy to cure type 2 diabetes [1, 2].

Obesity surgery is currently one of the most frequently performed surgical procedures in the US and Europe. The American Society of Bariatric Surgeons announced about 16,000 operations in the early 1990s and 103,000 procedures for the year 2003 [3]. Over the last four decades many different surgical techniques with various modifications have been published and named after the first-describing author. All procedures are based on the following three concepts:

(a) *Restrictive* surgery acts through a reduction of food intake by creating a small gastric reservoir and a narrow gastric outlet (e.g. vertical-banded gastroplasty or laparoscopic gastric banding).

(b) The *malabsorptive* procedure causes weight loss through restriction of nutritional absorption by reduced mucosal surface and shorter intestinal transit time (e.g. biliopancreatic diversion or duodenal switch).

(c) *Mixed* procedures combine both mechanisms (e.g. gastric bypass).

Each technique is associated with different outcomes and most importantly with treatment-specific short- and long-term complications. Therefore, it is essential for any surgical or nonsurgical speciality to understand which procedure is performed in an individual patient. The aim of this chapter is to discuss the most important and most commonly performed procedures with special emphasis on outcome and potential complications.

Epidemiology

Obesity is a growing health problem in many industrialized countries reaching epidemic proportions in Europe and the US [4]. One in five Americans has a BMI above 30 and 2.3% above 40 [5]. About 300,000 people per year die of causes related to their being overweight [6]. This proportion has only been exceeded by smoking. In 2003, approximately USD 3 billion was spent for bariatric surgical procedures. The situation in Europe is becoming comparable [7]. Not only is the adult population overweight, but also more and more children are above their ideal weight, e.g. 24% of 10-year-old boys in Switzerland and up to 30% in Italy are overweight [8]. This development is frightening since these overweight children have a high risk of becoming obese also as adults, with lesser chances for employment and social acceptance and significant health problems. These developments imply that the epidemic has just begun and future concepts are urgently needed to cope with this important issue.

History of Obesity Surgery

Obesity surgery was discovered as a result of gastric ulcer surgery when surgeons realized that patients after subtotal gastrectomy or after shortened gut lost weight. The first attempts in obesity surgery were made in the 1950s with the jejuno-ileal bypass procedures, where a significant part of the small bowel was bypassed and left in a blind loop. These procedures resulted in an excellent weight loss, but were associated with severe long-term complications such as electrolyte imbalance, nephrolithiasis, blind loop syndrome and cirrhosis [9, 10]. For many physicians the term 'bypass surgery' is still flawed with this unfavorable experience. This procedure has become obsolete and is not comparable with the current type of 'bypass surgery'. In 1966, Mason and Ito [11] developed the first gastric bypass, where a small gastric reservoir, so-called pouch, was created that was anastomosed to a jejunal loop. Afterwards, several modifications were developed [12, 13]. In 1977, a Roux-en-Y construction instead of a loop anastomosis was suggested [14]. This modification had the advantage of less anastomotic tension and no bile reflux through the stomach (fig. 2). With a Roux-en-Y construction, the option of variation of the limb length was possible and therefore the restrictive procedures were supplemented with a variable malabsorptive component (fig. 2). Randomized controlled trials have demonstrated that weight loss after gastric bypass procedure was comparable with that after jejuno-ileal bypass [14]. Therefore, the gastric bypass became the gold standard in bariatric surgery in the US for many years. In 1980, the vertical banded gastroplasty was developed as a purely restrictive procedure [15]. Weight reduction was achieved through a decrease of food intake by a small gastric reservoir and a small gastric outlet. Patients experienced satiety by the distension of the gastric pouch. The major advantage of this procedure was the intact passage through the whole intestinal tract.

With the rise of laparoscopic procedures, a new technique, purely restrictive as well, was developed in the 1990s in Europe, the so-called gastric banding [16]. The gastric banding neither cut nor stapled the stomach. In contrast to all other bariatric techniques, the diameter of the pouch outlet was adjustable through a port, which was placed in the subcutaneous tissue. In 1993, first reports demonstrated that this procedure was laparoscopically feasible [17, 18]. Since that time, gastric banding experienced a real boom in bariatric surgery because this procedure was simple, potentially fully reversible, effective, and easy to learn. However, due to the lack of long-term experience, laparoscopic gastric banding only got the FDA's approval in the US in the late 1990s. Therefore, most of the literature on long-term efficiency of gastric banding comes from Europe [17–24], whereas most bypass series are published from centers in the US [11, 25–32].

In addition to gastric bypass surgery, other purely malabsorbtive procedures were developed. These procedures originate from the jejuno-ileal bypass but with the important modification that no intestinal limb was without flow. The two most promising procedures were the biliopancreatic diversion by Scopinaro et al. [33] and the duodenal switch operation by Marceau et al. [34] altered to its current modification by Hess and Hess [31].

The latest revolution was the introduction of laparoscopic techniques in the late 1990s, which helped to promote this surgical treatment successfully. Nowadays, bariatric surgery is mainly performed by minimally invasive access surgery, with the advantage of better patient comfort and less wound complications [32, 35–42]. Open surgery should now be limited only to difficult revisional surgery.

Surgical Techniques

Indication and Selection of Patients

Patient selection and choosing the right procedure should always be assessed by an interdisciplinary team, considering all the possible questions and problems of the individual patient. This is additionally requested by many insurance companies [43].

The National Institutes of Health Consensus Development Conference on Gastrointestinal Surgery for Severe Obesity 1991 recommends [44–46]:

(1) Patients seeking therapy for severe obesity for the first time should be considered for treatment in a non-surgical program with integrated components of a dietary regimen, appropriate exercise, and behavioral modification and support.

(2) Gastric restrictive or bypass procedures could be considered for well-informed and motivated patients with acceptable operative risks.

(3) Patients who are candidates for surgical procedures should be selected carefully after evaluation by a multidisciplinary team with medical, surgical, psychiatric, and nutritional expertise.

(4) The operation should be performed by a surgeon substantially experienced with the appropriate procedures and working in a clinical setting with adequate support for all aspects of management and assessment.

(5) Lifelong medical surveillance after surgical therapy is a necessity.

The indications for bariatric surgery in adults (age >18 years) are well defined and are currently in most Western countries as follows [43–46; www.asbs.org]:

– BMI >40
    or
– BMI >35 with significant co-morbidities, e.g. cardiac disease, diabetes mellitus type 2, obstructive sleep apnea, hypertension, dyslipidemia, gastroesophageal reflux disease, stress urinary incontinence, arthritis of the weight bearing joints, infertility
    and
– (multiple) failure of dietary attempts at weight control.

Unfortunately, up to now there is only little evidence to select the best type of surgery for a specific patient. Often, the choice of procedure is driven by the surgeon's skills and local tradition (US vs. Europe) rather than by scientific evidence. However, there is some evidence that purely restrictive procedures should not be offered to patients with a BMI >50, since they might not lose enough weight to have a sufficient benefit from the procedure [47].

Patients with a BMI <50 might benefit from a less-invasive restrictive procedure such as gastric banding. Exclusion criteria for purely restrictive procedures are binge eating disorder, insufficient lower esophageal sphincter or esophageal dysmotility assessed by video fluoroscopic and manometric studies.

Patients who meet these exclusion criteria should be better treated with a mixed or purely malabsorbtive procedure such as gastric bypass or biliopancreatic diversion/duodenal switch procedure, respectively.

Furthermore, it has been shown that gastric bypass and duodenal switch procedures have a much better effect on the control of type 2 diabetes [2, 48]. Therefore, these operations are especially suitable for those with a BMI even lower than 50, and diabetes.

Surgical Technique

Patients are positioned in a 45° angle in a half-sitting position (beach-chair position). The pneumoperitoneum is applied by a closed Verress needle approach and 5–6 trokars are usually inserted.

Laparoscopic Gastric Banding (fig. 1)

In this procedure, a tunnel behind the cardia of the stomach is created after calibration of the small gastric pouch of 15–25 ml. Afterwards, the band is positioned around the stomach through the created tunnel and locked. On the anterior wall the band is covered with a fundic wrap which is fixed with several nonabsorbable sutures to avoid gastric herniation. On the posterior side the band is fixed by surrounding tissue. The band is connected to a reservoir which is placed in the subcutaneous tissue enabling later diameter adjustment of the band. The day after surgery, Gastrographine™ examination is routinely performed to document the correct band position and to detect gastric leakage. Thereafter, the patient is started on a fluid diet which is steadily increased to normal food over the next 2–3 weeks. Patients are usually discharged on the first postoperative day. Four to six weeks after surgery the band is inflated for the first time.

Laparoscopic Gastric Bypass (fig. 2)

The first step is the creation of a small gastric pouch by transecting the stomach with a stapler. Thereafter, the jejunum is transected 50 cm distal to the duodeno-jejunal flexure. The distal jejunum is brought up in an antecolic position to the pouch and anastomosed with a 25-mm diameter circular stapler. The jejuno-jejunostomy is constructed as a Roux-en-Y limb. The alimentary limb is 150 cm for a 'long limb' gastric bypass and 75 cm for a 'short limb' gastric bypass [30]. A distal gastric bypass is defined when the level of the jejuno-jejunostomy

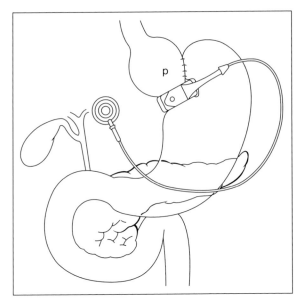

Fig. 1. Laparoscopic gastric banding procedure with a proximal pouch (p). The subcutaneous reservoir allows one to adjust the diameter of the stoma between the pouch and the remnant stomach.

results in a common channel length of 100 cm [49]. Patients start with liquid diet after a Gastrographine™ swallow examination on the third postoperative day has excluded leakage. Patients are usually discharged 5 days after surgery.

Biliopancreatic Diversion/Duodenal Switch (fig. 3)

A tube-like stomach with a volume of about 250 ml is created by resecting the greater curvature. The duodenum is transected distal to the pylorus. The small intestine is divided 250 cm prior to the ileocecal valve and the distal part is anastomosed to the postpyloric duodenum. The proximal small intestine is reanastomosed to the distal ileum 100 cm from the ileocecal valve as a Roux-en-Y construction.

The biliopancreatic diversion after Scopinaro follows the same principal; however, in this technique the stomach is dissected horizontally, the distal stomach is totally removed and the common channel is shortened to 50 cm. Of note, in both procedures the reduction of the gastric volume does not lead to a food restriction but to a reduction of acid-producing parietal cells to avoid anastomotic ulcers. The early postoperative follow-up of both procedures is similar to that of a bypass procedure. However, the malabsorbtive nature of this procedure requires a careful long-term follow-up to control vitamin (especially vitamin B

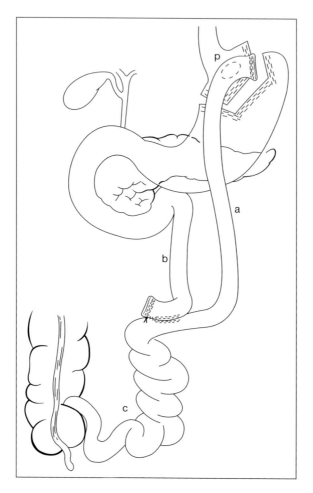

Fig. 2. The proximal gastric bypass consists of a small pouch (p) of about 25 ml to which the alimentary limb (a) of 150 cm is connected. The biliary limb (b) that measures 50 cm is connected to the alimentary limb as a Roux-en-Y construction. The length of the common channel (c) is variable. The distal gastric bypass has a common channel length of 100 cm and the alimentary limb is variable.

complexes) and mineral levels (especially ferrum and calcium) and it requires a good patient compliance.

Mechanism and Outcome of the Different Procedures

The laparoscopic gastric banding procedure leads to a restriction of food intake. The average patient loses 40–60% of the excess weight within 2 years after surgery. This corresponds to a BMI reduction by 10–12 points [19–22, 50, 51].

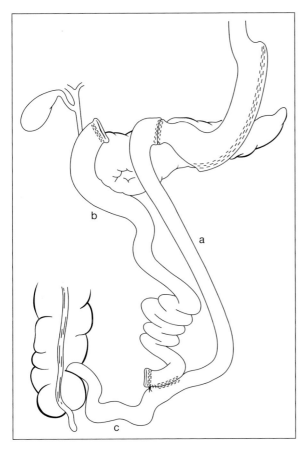

Fig. 3. In the duodenal switch operation the greater curvature of the stomach is resected and the volume of the gastric remnant is 250–300 ml. The alimentary limb (a) is anastomosed to the proximal duodenum and measures 150 cm. The biliary limb (b) is variable and the common channel (c) has a length of 100 cm.

However, experience in laparoscopic gastric banding has shown a high rate of long-term failures and complications. For example, band erosions, band slippages and esophageal dilatation have been reported in 15–58% [19, 23, 52, 53]. In the long-term, pouch dilatations and esophageal dysmotility occur in up to 40% [24; Weber et al., unpubl. data] and can lead to failure of the system requiring a redo operation in up to 20% [54, 55].

The gastric bypass procedure generates a moderate restriction of the food intake in combination with malabsorbtive mechanisms. The food in the alimentary limb is separated from the digestive juices (produced by pancreas and liver), which is transported by the biliary limb. Both, food and digestive juices including bile are merged in the common channel where full digestion and absorption occurs. Additionally, the gastric bypass induces a suppression of gastrointestinal hormones, such as plasma ghrelin [56]. Moreover, thus far unknown mechanisms produce a dramatic improvement of diabetes, even before other significant weight reduction [2, 57].

Patients after gastric bypass lose 69–77% of their excess weight within 24 months [26, 28, 29, 58]. In a distal gastric bypass with a more distal level of the jejuno-jejunostomy, weight loss can even amount up to 90% of the excess weight [49]. Patients often suffer on vitamin B_{12} and iron deficiency after gastric bypass. Therefore, careful follow-up is mandatory to ensure adequate vitamin B_{12} and iron levels following supplementary therapy.

Studies comparing bypass versus banding procedures have demonstrated that bypass procedures are superior to gastric banding in terms of weight loss and correction of hypertension and type 2 diabetes [59, 60; Weber et al., unpubl. data]. Bypass procedures are associated with more early complications, while gastric banding has more late complications which require re-operations, mostly a conversion to gastric bypass [Weber et al., unpubl. data]. Recent data on large series with laparoscopic gastric bypass surgery report a perioperative mortality rate of 0.5% [25, 28] compared to 0.05% for laparoscopic gastric banding [37].

The biliopancreatic diversion/duodenal switch operation acts through malabsorbtive mechanisms similar to the gastric bypass. Patients have almost no restriction of food intake [61]. The procedure has similar perioperative morbidity rates in comparison to gastric bypass. The reduction of excess weight by 64–74% is also comparable to gastric bypass procedures [27, 31, 62]. On the other hand, patients with biliopancreatic diversion usually pass 3–4 stools per day. Diarrhea is observed in up to 14% and up to 43% of the patients report unpleasant odor of stools and flatus as a major problem [27]. Equivalent to the gastric bypass procedure, comorbidities are influenced in a positive manner, when type 2 diabetes disappears and hypertension as well as other comorbidities decrease significantly.

Secondary Procedures

The increased numbers of performed bariatric operations (>103,000 per year in 2003!) [3] will also result in an increase of complications which may require surgical revisions or secondary procedures. As more than 70,000 patients have received a gastric banding procedure over the past decade worldwide, it can be predicted that we will see many patients requiring rescue procedures like conversion to gastric bypass [23].

Pouch complications including band slippage are the most common reasons for failure of a gastric banding procedure. The theoretic options to treat this failure are removal or reposition of the band [53, 63] or conversion to another bariatric procedure [54]. Enlarged concentric pouches or eccentric pouches [24, 64] due to band slippage can lead to an acute gastric obstruction. This condition can be an indication for an emergency operation especially when the patient suffers from continuous abdominal pain accompanied by tachycardia, tachypnea, or fever. These dangerous symptoms might indicate gastric necrosis of the slipped stomach [65]. Simple removal of the silicone band without replacement usually corrects the slippage-related complications, but it is associated with rapid recurrence or persistence of obesity.

Laparoscopic gastric band repositioning or rebanding have been described as possible rescue procedures. However, only few data regarding these procedures are published, and show disappointing results [54, 63].

Gastric rebanding is an option for patients with successful and stable weight loss after banding [66] unless there are new contraindications for this restrictive procedure such as esophageal dysmotility or reflux. If a purely restrictive procedure failed, it should not be repeated [54].

The laparoscopic or open conversion to a gastric bypass has also been proposed to enable effective control of obesity [55, 67], especially in the light of the above-mentioned contraindications for a rebanding procedure [23, 68].

The conversion to a bypass is a very challenging operation that can be performed laparoscopically. It has been shown that rebanding is inferior to conversion to a bypass procedure in terms of weight loss (within 2 years after secondary surgery) [54].

It is very rare that a previous bypass procedure leads to a re-operation due to insufficient weight loss. However, in those cases with insufficient weight loss the size of the proximal gastric pouch has to be re-evaluated firstly. An enlarged pouch can be reduced laparoscopically to restore the restrictive effect of the gastric bypass. In case of a correct pouch size, the enhancement of the malabsorbtive effect by shortening of the common channel laparoscopically should be considered [49, 69]. On the other hand, if patients lose too much weight with severe vitamin and iron deficiencies it is possible to lengthen the common channel to increase the absorptive surface of the bowel.

Psychological Aspect from the Surgeon's Point of View

Morbid obese patients have a higher prevalence of mental disorders, especially eating disorders (e.g. 27–65% binge eating disorder) [70], see also chapter on the epidemiology of binge eating disorder by Hilbert [this vol., pp. 149–164]. Furthermore, the prevalence of psychological problems is also higher compared to the normal weight population [71–74]. However, many of these mental disorders are due to reactive depression, which is a result of the overweight [71].

The psychological aspects are important for surgeons regarding the indication for obesity surgery, choice of procedure and follow-up. Patients with personality disorders seem to have different grades of success if they are confronted with conservative or operative treatment [75]. It has been shown that surgical procedures can positively influence eating disorders [76]. However, patients have to be in stable psychological conditions to be enrolled (or included) into a surgical bariatric program. Patients with anxiety and high psychological stress scales in the Psychosocial Stress and Symptom Questionnaire (PSSQ) should not be excluded from bariatric surgery. This is supported by a study [77], where patients with preoperative high stress scales preoperatively decreased their values after bariatric surgery whereas patients who were rejected or withdrew their consent maintained high stress values and showed a worse outcome with significantly more consultations of physicians.

Even patients with severe mental disorders such as psychotic episodes experience an improvement of their psychological well-being after successful bariatric surgery as long as a caring psychiatrist supports the surgical treatment [78–80]. Therefore, patients with stable psychiatric disease can be treated with a bariatric procedure. However, the type of procedure may be influenced by the psychological disorders since some eating disorders, such as binge eating disorders, are not good indications for a purely restrictive procedure. Binge eaters do not realize their satiety and therefore use their esophagus as a reservoir leading to long-term esophageal damage [54]. On the other hand, some authors believe that binge eating disorders can disappear after bypass surgery [81].

Outlook

The ongoing epidemic development of obesity is a great challenge for the society at the present as well as in the future. Surgeons and physicians have to develop concepts to cope with the increasing number of obese patients. This is not only restricted to health problems but also has a great impact on society. Concepts have to be developed to keep the manpower of these individuals and to minimize costs of the national health services.

Obesity surgery is not yet fully accepted by many members of society. This has to change since morbidity and costs arising from obesity reach the same proportions as cancer and cardiovascular disease in modern societies.

Future concepts might even include specialized institutions that manage obesity in an interdisciplinary approach. It is our strong belief that the involvement of each specialist is of paramount importance.

Psychological evaluation is already an essential part of the preoperative work-up. This allows us to identify patients who are at risk for decompensation who could be enrolled into accompanying psychotherapy. More work will have to be done finding the patient who will profit best from a purely restrictive procedure and supporting the patient to cope with the infinity of the bypass procedure.

To select the best approach for the individual patient will be one of the focuses of future surgical research. Although obesity surgery is expanding dramatically, many of the procedures are not yet standardized (e.g. limb length of gastric bypass) and procedures are not yet compared to each other in a randomized controlled trial. Bariatric procedures themselves differ very much from center to center and even among surgeons. Gold standards will have to be established and indications have to be more tailored to the individual patient and should not depend on the technical skills of the surgeon.

Surgeons will have to manage more late complications and secondary failures of first procedures. Plastic surgeons will have to deal with the sequelae of extensive weight loss.

Many of the principles of bariatric surgical procedures are not yet understood, enterohumoral and central nervous feedback mechanisms are still unknown. Future research on this issue should help for the individual selection of the surgical bariatric procedure. Whether bariatric surgical procedures will be extended for purely co-morbidity-related indications such as diabetes mellitus [82] without the presence of obesity will be discussed.

Furthermore, physicians and surgeons have to take obesity in childhood seriously since there is a dramatic increase of prevalence in most western countries. Conservative treatment concepts often fail in children as in adults in the long term [83]. Therefore, surgical concepts in adolescence will emerge and might even have a greater potential since eating habits are not fully developed in these individuals [84, 85].

Finally the reimbursement of surgical therapies has to be re-evaluated. Costs of surgical procedures have to be balanced in terms of long-term cost of threatening co-morbidities such as coronary heart disease or diabetes. Unfortunately, the increasing cost pressure forces health insurance companies to be more and more restrictive. This results in incoherent decision-making and in some cases even in discrimination of obese patients by withholding them from adequate surgical treatment.

References

1   Brolin RE: Update: NIH consensus conference. Gastrointestinal surgery for severe obesity. Nutrition 1996;12:403–404.
2   Pories WJ, et al: Who would have thought it? An operation proves to be the most effective therapy for adult-onset diabetes mellitus. Ann Surg 1995;222:339–350; discussion 350–352.
3   Steinbrook R: Surgery for severe obesity. N Engl J Med 2004;350:1075–1079.

4   World Health Organization: Obesity-Prevention and Managing the Global Epidemic. Report of a WHO Consultation on Obesity. Geneva, WHO, 1997.

5   Mokdad AH, et al: Prevalence of obesity, diabetes, and obesity-related health risk factors, 2001. JAMA 2003;289:76–79.

6   Allison DB, et al: Annual deaths attributable to obesity in the United States. JAMA 1999;282: 1530–1538.

7   Obesity: Preventing and managing the global epidemic. Report of a WHO consultation. World Health Organ Tech Rep Ser 2000;894:i–xii, 1–253.

8   Bellizzi MC: Prevalence of childhood and adolescent overweight and obesity in Asian and European countries; in Chen C, Dietz WH (eds): Obesity in Childhood and Adolescence. Nestec Ltd., Vevey, Switzerland. Philadelphia, Lippincott Williams & Wilkins, 2002.

9   Gianetta E, et al: 2 cases of death caused by hepatic insufficiency after jejuno-ileal bypass for obesity. Minerva Chir 1979;34:1087–1096.

10   Buchwald HR, Rucker RD: The rise and fall of jejunoileal bypass; in Nelson RL, Nyhus LM (eds): surgery of the small intestine. Norwalk, Appleton Century Crofts, 1987, pp 529–541.

11   Mason EE, Ito C: Gastric bypass in obesity. Surg Clin N Am 1967;47:1345–1351.

12   Alden JF: Gastric and jejunoileal bypass. A comparison in the treatment of morbid obesity. Arch Surg 1977;112:799–806.

13   Torres JC, Oca CF, Garrison RN: Gastric bypass: Roux-en-Y gastrojejunostomy from the lesser curvature. South Med J 1983;76:1217–1221.

14   Griffen WO Jr., Young VL, Stevenson CC: A prospective comparison of gastric and jejunoileal bypass procedures for morbid obesity. Ann Surg 1977;186:500–509.

15   Mason EE: Vertical banded gastroplasty for obesity. Arch Surg 1982;117:701–706.

16   Kuzmak LI: A review of seven years' experience with silicone gastric banding. Obes Surg 1991;1:403–408.

17   Belachew M, et al: Laparoscopic adjustable silicone gastric banding in the treatment of morbid obesity. A preliminary report. Surg Endosc 1994;8:1354–1356.

18   Forsell P, Hallberg D, Hellers G: Gastric banding for morbid obesity: Initial experience with a new adjustable band. Obes Surg 1993;3:369–374.

19   Suter M, et al: A 3-year experience with laparoscopic gastric banding for obesity. Surg Endosc 2000;14:532–536.

20   Miller K, Hell E: Laparoscopic adjustable gastric banding: A prospective 4-year follow-up study. Obes Surg 1999;9:183–187.

21   Dargent J: Laparoscopic adjustable gastric banding: Lessons from the first 500 patients in a single institution. Obes Surg 1999;9:446–452.

22   Zinzindohoue F, et al: Laparoscopic gastric banding: A minimally invasive surgical treatment for morbid obesity: Prospective study of 500 consecutive patients. Ann Surg 2003;237:1–9.

23   Gustavsson S, Westling A: Laparoscopic adjustable gastric banding: Complications and side effects responsible for the poor long-term outcome. Semin Laparosc Surg 2002;9:115–124.

24   Peternac D, et al: The effects of laparoscopic adjustable gastric banding on the proximal pouch and the esophagus. Obes Surg 2001;11:76–86.

25   Higa KD, Boone KB, Ho T: Complications of the laparoscopic Roux-en-Y gastric bypass: 1,040 patients – What have we learned? Obes Surg 2000;10:509–513.

26   Wittgrove AC, Clark GW: Laparoscopic gastric bypass, Roux-en-Y-500 patients: Technique and results, with 3–60 month follow-up. Obes Surg 2000;10:233–239.

27   Marceau P, et al: Biliopancreatic diversion with duodenal switch. World J Surg 1998;22:947–954.

28   Schauer PR, et al: Outcomes after laparoscopic Roux-en-Y gastric bypass for morbid obesity. Ann Surg 2000;232:515–529.

29   DeMaria EJ, et al: Results of 281 consecutive total laparoscopic Roux-en-Y gastric bypasses to treat morbid obesity. Ann Surg 2002;235:640–645; discussion 645–647.

30   Brolin RE, et al: Long-limb gastric bypass in the superobese. A prospective randomized study. Ann Surg 1992;215:387–395.

31   Hess DS, Hess DW: Biliopancreatic diversion with a duodenal switch. Obes Surg 1998;8:267–282.

32   Nguyen NT, et al: Laparoscopic versus open gastric bypass: A randomized study of outcomes, quality of life, and costs. Ann Surg 2001;234:279–289; discussion 289–291.

33 Scopinaro N, et al: Bilio-pancreatic bypass for obesity: II. Initial experience in man. Br J Surg 1979;66:618–620.

34 Marceau P, et al: Biliopancreatic diversion with a new type of gastrectomy. Obes Surg 1993;3: 29–35.

35 Sundbom M, Gustavsson S: Randomized clinical trial of hand-assisted laparoscopic versus open Roux-en-Y gastric bypass for the treatment of morbid obesity. Br J Surg 2004;91:418–423.

36 Westling A, Gustavsson S: Laparoscopic vs open Roux-en-Y gastric bypass: A prospective, randomized trial. Obes Surg 2001;11:284–292.

37 Chapman AE, et al: Laparoscopic adjustable gastric banding in the treatment of obesity: A systematic literature review. Surgery 2004;135:326–351.

38 Schauer PR: Open and laparoscopic surgical modalities for the management of obesity. J Gastrointest Surg 2003;7:468–475.

39 Kim WW, et al: Laparoscopic vs. open biliopancreatic diversion with duodenal switch: A comparative study. J Gastrointest Surg 2003;7:552–557.

40 Courcoulas A, et al: Comparing the outcomes after laparoscopic versus open gastric bypass: A matched paired analysis. Obes Surg 2003;13:341–346.

41 Courcoulas A, et al: The relationship of surgeon and hospital volume to outcome after gastric bypass surgery in Pennsylvania: A 3-year summary. Surgery 2003;134:613–621; discussion 621–623.

42 Lujan JA, Frutos MD, Hernandez Q, Liron R, Cuenca JR, Valero G, Parrilla P: Laparoscopic versus open gastric bypass in the treatment of morbid obesity: A randomized prospective study. Ann Surg 2004;239:433–437.

43 Bundesgesetz über die Krankenversicherung der Schweizerischen Eidgenossenschaft. Anhang 1 des Artikels 1 der Leistungsverordnung (in Kraft ab 1.1.2000).

44 Hubbard VS, Hall WH: Gastrointestinal surgery for severe obesity. Obes Surg 1991;1:257–265.

45 Gastrointestinal surgery for severe obesity: National Institutes of Health Consensus Development Conference Statement. Am J Clin Nutr 1992;55:615S–619S.

46 Gastrointestinal surgery for severe obesity. Consens Statement 1991;9:1–20.

47 Buchwald H: A bariatric surgery algorithm. Obes Surg 2002;12:733–746; discussion 747–750.

48 Cowan GS, Jr., Buffington CK: Significant changes in blood pressure, glucose, and lipids with gastric bypass surgery. World J Surg 1998;22:987–992.

49 Torres JC: Why I prefer gastric bypass distal Roux-en-Y gastroileostomy. Obes Surg 1991;1: 189–194.

50 Dixon JB, Dixon ME, O'Brien PE: Pre-operative predictors of weight loss at 1-year after Lap-Band surgery. Obes Surg 2001;11:200–207.

51 O'Brien PE, et al: Prospective study of a laparoscopically placed, adjustable gastric band in the treatment of morbid obesity. Br J Surg 1999;86:113–118.

52 Holeczy P, Novak P, Kralova A: 30% complications with adjustable gastric banding: What did we do wrong? Obes Surg 2001;11:748–751.

53 Niville E, Dams A: Late pouch dilation after laparoscopic adjustable gastric and esophagogastric banding: Incidence, treatment, and outcome. Obes Surg 1999;9:381–384.

54 Weber M, et al: Laparoscopic Roux-en-Y gastric bypass, but not rebanding, should be proposed as rescue procedure for patients with failed laparoscopic gastric banding. Ann Surg 2003;238: 827–833; discussion 833–834.

55 Westling A, Ohrvall M, Gustavsson S: Roux-en-Y gastric bypass after previous unsuccessful gastric restrictive surgery. J Gastrointest Surg 2002;6:206–211.

56 Cummings DE, et al: Plasma ghrelin levels after diet-induced weight loss or gastric bypass surgery. N Engl J Med 2002;346:1623–1630.

57 Rubino F, Gagner M: Potential of surgery for curing type 2 diabetes mellitus. Ann Surg 2002;236: 554–559.

58 Higa KD, et al: Laparoscopic Roux-en-Y gastric bypass for morbid obesity: Technique and preliminary results of our first 400 patients. Arch Surg 2000;135:1029–1033; discussion 1033–1034.

59 Schauer PR, et al: Effect of laparoscopic Roux-en Y gastric bypass on type 2 diabetes mellitus. Ann Surg 2003;238:467–484; discussion 84–85.

60 Sugerman HJ, et al: Diabetes and hypertension in severe obesity and effects of gastric bypass-induced weight loss. Ann Surg 2003;237:751–756; discussion 757–758.

---

61 Anthone GJ, et al: The duodenal switch operation for the treatment of morbid obesity. Ann Surg 2003;238:618–627; discussion 627–628.
62 Ren CJ, Patterson E, Gagner M: Early results of laparoscopic biliopancreatic diversion with duodenal switch: A case series of 40 consecutive patients. Obes Surg 2000;10:514–523; discussion 524.
63 Suter M: Laparoscopic band repositioning for pouch dilatation/slippage after gastric banding: Disappointing results. Obes Surg 2001;11:507–512.
64 Spivak H, Favretti F: Avoiding postoperative complications with the LAP-BAND system. Am J Surg 2002;184:31S–37S.
65 Methods for Voluntary Weight Loss and Control. Proceedings of NIH Technology Assessment Conference. Bethesda, Maryland, 30 March–1 April 1992. Ann Intern Med 1993;119:641–770.
66 Weiss HG, et al: Surgical revision after failure of laparoscopic adjustable gastric banding. Br J Surg 2004;91:235–241.
67 Gawdat K: Bariatric re-operations: Are they preventable? Obes Surg 2000;10:525–529.
68 Balsiger BM, et al: Gastroesophageal reflux after intact vertical banded gastroplasty: Correction by conversion to Roux-en-Y gastric bypass. J Gastrointest Surg 2000;4:276–281.
69 Fobi MA, et al: Revision of failed gastric bypass to distal Roux-en-Y gastric bypass: A review of 65 cases. Obes Surg 2001;11:190–195.
70 Adami GF, Gandolfo P, Scopinaro N: Binge eating in obesity. Int J Obes Relat Metab Disord 1996;20:793–794.
71 Lang T, et al: Psychological comorbidity and quality of life of patients with morbid obesity and requesting gastric banding. Schweiz Med Wochenschr 2000;130:739–748.
72 Saunders R: Binge eating in gastric bypass patients before surgery. Obes Surg 1999;9:72–76.
73 Becker ES, et al: Obesity and mental illness in a representative sample of young women. Int J Obes Relat Metab Disord 2001;25:S5–S9.
74 Black DW, Goldstein RB, Mason EE: Prevalence of mental disorder in 88 morbidly obese bariatric clinic patients. Am J Psychiatry 1992;149:227–234.
75 Berman WH, et al: The effect of psychiatric disorders on weight loss in obesity clinic patients. Behav Med 1993;18:167–172.
76 Lang T, et al: Impact of gastric banding on eating behavior and weight. Obes Surg 2002;12: 100–107.
77 Buddeberg-Fischer B, Klaghofer R, Sigrist S, Buddeberg C: Impact of psychosocial stress and symptoms on indication for bariatric surgery and outcome in morbidly obese patients. Obes Surg 2003;14:361–369.
78 Schok M, et al: Quality of life after laparoscopic adjustable gastric banding for severe obesity: Postoperative and retrospective preoperative evaluations. Obes Surg 2000;10:502–508.
79 Powers PS, et al: Outcome of gastric restriction procedures: Weight, psychiatric diagnoses, and satisfaction. Obes Surg 1997;7:471–477.
80 Adami GF, et al: Body image in obese patients before and after stable weight reduction following bariatric surgery. J Psychosom Res 1999;46:275–281.
81 Adami GF, et al: Body image in binge eating disorder. Obes Surg 1998;8:517–519.
82 Rubino F, Marescaux J: Effect of duodenal-jejunal exclusion in a non-obese animal model of type 2 diabetes: A new perspective for an old disease. Ann Surg 2004;239:1–11.
83 Epstein LH, et al: Do children lose and maintain weight easier than adults: A comparison of child and parent weight changes from six months to ten years. Obes Res 1995;3:411–417.
84 Dolan K, et al: Laparoscopic gastric banding in morbidly obese adolescents. Obes Surg 2003;13: 101–104.
85 Sugerman HJ, et al: Bariatric surgery for severely obese adolescents. J Gastrointest Surg 2003;7: 102–107; discussion 107–108.

PD Dr. Markus Weber
Division for Visceral and Transplantation Surgery
University Hospital, Rämistrasse 100, CH–8091 Zurich (Switzerland)
Tel. +41 1 255 3868, Fax +41 1 255 8941, E-Mail markus.weber@usz.ch

Munsch S, Beglinger C (eds): Obesity and Binge Eating Disorder.
Bibl Psychiatr. Basel, Karger, 2005, No 171, pp 117–137

Treatment of Obese Children

Caroline Braet

Department of Developmental, Personality and Social Psychology,
Ghent University, Ghent, Belgium

Childhood and adolescent obesity has increased dramatically over the past 25 years. The prevalence of overweight doubled among children 6–11 years of age and tripled among those 12–17 years of age. Approximately 26–31% of American children and about 14–22% of European children are overweight, when overweight is defined by the NHES as the 85th percentile of BMI [1]. Taking the 95th percentile of BMI, about 9–13% of the children are obese [1, 2]. The prevalence of obesity among children has never reached before such epidemic proportions as today [3].

Overweight in childhood can no longer be considered a benign condition or one related only to appearance. Pediatric obesity increases the risk of adult obesity [4] and, long-standing obesity is associated with health risks in adults [5]. Furthermore, childhood obesity is associated with health complications, including elevated blood pressure, hyperinsulinemia and glucose intolerance, and respiratory abnormalities [3, 6]. The effects of childhood obesity on morbidity and mortality suggest that effective prevention and intervention for childhood obesity is recommended.

For decades now 'going on a diet' is considered the ultimate solution to lose excess weight. Unfortunately, time and again it turns out that weight is regained after the dietary treatment period and that people sometimes weigh more than before [7]. Moreover, going on a diet is believed to have harmful side effects, such as an increased risk of developing binge eating and disorders in the regulation of the basal metabolism [8]. Scientific research came to the conclusion that there is no proper treatment method for obese adults today and that there are only a few 'promising' treatment goals [7]: (1) aiming at weight management instead of weight loss, with a maximum of 10% weight loss allowed; (2) establishing a healthy lifestyle, which implies a more favorable prognosis with respect to the prevention of diseases, and (3) the prevention of overweight, e.g. through early intervention in obese children.

In order to be able to give a good idea of the treatment of childhood obesity, this chapter will successively deal with the biological and psychological models to explain for the onset of child obesity, therapy indications and the current treatment.

Onset of Childhood Obesity: The Biological Model

There is a clear consensus about the etiology of obesity and the mechanism of the development of obesity is identical in children and in adults. Obesity refers to an excess accumulation of body fat as a result of an imbalance between energy intake and energy expenditure [9]. When the energy intake exceeds the physical requirements, the excess energy is in some people converted into fat, which may in time produce fat reserves and lead to obesity.

The causes of a disturbed balance in overweight people are multifactorial, with changes in energy intake and expenditure related to both subtle and obvious movements in societal behavioral habits. US studies show positive correlation between television viewing and overweight [10]. Energy expenditure has been reduced by an increase in sedentary activities, a decrease in the need to expend energy in daily routines, and an increase in the use of cars and other forms of transport. On a related level, the safety of the environment can encourage or discourage a child from being physically active [11]. Furthermore, food is now more attractive, promoted and simply obtained. Especially energy-dense foods are plentiful and relatively inexpensive. These factors may be especially pertinent for families living in lower socio-economic strata, where limited financial constraints may favor purchasing less expensive yet more fattening foods. However, dietary intake during childhood is difficult to measure and its predictive value for adiposity is unclear [12].

To attribute obesity solely to eating habits or low levels of exercises, would be a gross generalization. Studies with twins and adopted children demonstrated that there is a genetic 'susceptibility' to developing obesity. The genetic factors have recently received much attention in medical circles as well as in the lay press after the discovery of the leptin gene. At the moment already dozens of gene fractions have been found, which all together can account for up to 30% of the variance [13, 14]. The more obese gene fractions you have, the greater the chance of developing obesity. This partial clarification of the genetic factors that influence the development of overweight has so far not led to therapeutic options. In view of the diversity of the genetic factors, it is not very likely that this will change in the near future. The geneticist Bouchard also indicates that overweight can only be revealed if someone is put in a situation of personal overfeeding for some time. This is hopeful for the treatment of childhood

---

obesity: it is mainly a question of searching, together with the patient, a balance between energy intake and energy expenditure and in this way preventing further overfeeding.

Psychological Explanations for the Onset of Childhood Obesity

Psychological explanation models are still subject of discussion. Research should first and foremost focus on contextual factors with respect to eating behavior [7].

The externality theory persisted for a long time [15]. According to this model, obese children have an increased responsiveness to food and this is seen as the consequence of a personality trait, called 'externality'. A typical study from the seventies is the experiment of Rodin and Slochower [16] with 107 girls between the ages of 9 and 15. In a holiday camp there was plenty of food for 8 weeks. The children were allowed to eat without restraint to their heart's content. The girls that scored high for 'externality' afterwards clearly appeared to have gained more weight than the other girls. The externality hypothesis was subject to severe criticism. With respect to obesity, it did not sufficiently demonstrate universality or the causal relationship.

Behavior therapy put forward the assumption that obese people have developed bad eating habits, such as eating in the car, in front of the television, at work, when feeling alone. Consequently, too many situations are associated with 'eating', which could explain the susceptibility of obese children to external food factors. The treatment resulting from this assumption consists in learning techniques derived from self-regulation exercises, such as restriction of the number of eating situations.

Meanwhile, Schlundt et al. [17] demonstrated that obese people can display at least 5 different eating behaviors over a period of 2 weeks, i.e. healthy eating habits, strict food restraint, dietary behavior alternated with binge eating, emotional eating and unrestricted overeating. So, eating behavior is more complex than initially thought and each of these eating patterns is now still subject of research.

Emotional eating is not studied extensively, although recent work by Goodman and Whitaker [18] showed that depressive mood predicted obesity at follow-up, after controlling for other variables. Braet and Van Strien [19] already demonstrated a positive correlation between emotional eating and overweight in obese children and Pine et al. [20] found in a longitudinal study a significant relationship between psychiatric problems and subsequent increased BMI in young adulthood, especially in females.

The boundary model of Herman and Polivy [21] was brought forward as an explanation model for 'overeating' in adults and recently in children as well. On the basis of observations and experimental research, this model describes that it is impossible to constantly maintain a diet and that this at times inevitably leads to a relapse in the form of an uncontrolled binge-eating episode. In this model, it is further assumed that people that are frequently on a diet have moved their biological limits with respect to hunger and satiety and have replaced them by a cognitive dietary limit. The chance of failure increases as the diet is stricter or if one is emotional, since the imposed self-regulation is then more and more put to the test. This would mean that overweight people that are on a diet will paradoxically have increasingly more problems with 'overeating'. Although this model mainly holds out in explanation of bulimia nervosa [22], it is assumed that it can explain also the eating problems of some obese people [23].

More and more obese people appear to form a heterogeneous group. This heterogeneity has implications for the treatment: It seems, for example, wise to distinguish between obese people that do/do not suffer from binge eating (the so-called binge eaters), those that are/are not on a diet (the restrainers) and those that indulge/do not indulge in emotional eating, in adults as well as in children [24]. Anyway, it also seems advisable not to put children on a strict diet.

The role of the parents and the family in the development and maintenance of the eating habits of children still has to be investigated further. Very useful in this respect are the findings of Leann Birch. Food is often used by parents to reinforce desired or undesired behavior. Parents rewarding their children with sweets increase the attractiveness of sweets in general [25]. Several studies also indicated that parents can encourage their children to eat [26]. Especially eating 'more' and 'longer' can be learned in this way. Without parental intervention, the chance that a toddler eats is about 1 of 2; with parental intervention this chance increases to 3 of 4. Specific interactions between parents and children also explain other forms of learned behavior such as always finishing one's plate, asking for a second portion because one wants to be a big girl or boy, etc. Although it seems reasonable to assume that the eating style of obese children is the result of former reinforcing processes during family meals, only recently studies in obese children emerge. Drucker et al. [27] showed that mothers influence their child's eating behavior; the rates of food offers and total prompts were significantly related to the child's rate of calorie intake, and the time spent eating by the child. Furthermore, Leasle et al. [28] demonstrated that obese children indeed ate faster and with larger bites during a standardized experimental meal in their laboratory, only when the mother was present.

Finally, delay of the fulfilment of one's needs, tolerance of hunger, dealing with frustrations and resistance against food persuaders are self-regulation skills that are gradually acquired through education and learning. Within this context, permanent eating may also be considered as a behavior deficit, not (yet) having learned good eating habits. In some obese children, the lack of control over food may be situated within a general lack of self-regulation skills. The parents of these children often find it difficult to set clear limits and to make concrete arrangements with their child. In such cases, the treatment for overweight necessarily implies acting on the parenting skills.

Psychological Consequences of Obesity

Obese people are, on the basis of their appearance, stigmatized as being unattractive, stupid, lazy or unfriendly [29]. Moreover, the environment often considers obese people as being fully responsible for their condition [30], which provokes antipathy with others [31]. As a consequence, obese youngsters often have fewer friends, which can interfere with the development of their social skills [3]. Another implication is the fact that obese children are often considered as being more mature than they really are, which can lead to feelings of not being able to come up to the expectations of the environment [3].

Several studies examined whether and how the above-mentioned consequences can influence the self-perception of obese youngsters. Dietz [3] concludes that younger obese children still have positive self-perceptions. The development of their self-concept is merely based upon the feedback of their parents. Older children, on the other hand, for whom peers and society become more important, have more chance of developing negative self-perceptions. Here, several authors [32–34] state that, on the basis of a multidimensional model of the self-concept, especially those components of the self-perception related to overweight and to social interactions become negatively influenced.

Overweight during adolescence has been related to concerns about shape and eating [35, 36]. Especially obese children presenting for a treatment of obesity, display a higher prevalence of psychological problems than obese children not seeking treatment [32]. The children that seek treatment show a lower self-esteem and more general psychopathology. In a study assessing child functioning, approximately half of the sample of the children, presenting for a weight loss treatment, were found to have elevated scores on at least one scale of the Child Behavior Checklist [37], which means: more emotional and behavioral problems, more depression.

The psychological burden for children with enduring overweight is significant and can lead to depression and social isolation [38, 39]. Body-related stigmata influence the social interactions between people. Consequently, obese persons are less loved, are often neglected, laughed at or teased [29]. This can affect other domains of their lives as well. Once they become young adults, obese people seem to receive less higher education, earn less money and marry to a lesser extent [40, 41].

Berkowitz et al. [42] observed symptoms of binge eating in about 30% of adolescent obese girls who sought weight reduction. Similar findings were found by Decaluwé et al. [43]. Obese children and adolescents who report binge eating show higher levels of eating pathology and lower self-esteem. The marked difference between obese children with and without binge eating suggests the need for specific interventions for obese binge eaters [see also chapter by Munsch and Hilbert, this vol., pp. 180–196].

Treatment of Obese Children: Current Views

In the overview by Jelalian and Saelens [44] on 'evidence-based' treatments for obese children, published in the *Journal of Pediatric Psychology*, it has been demonstrated that an effective treatment must always occur within a behavioral-therapeutic framework. These researchers examined 61 studies on obesity, 42 of which met the label of 'good research'. Reviews of the characteristics of childhood obesity treatment studies are presented also by Epstein et al. [45] and Goldfried et al. [46].

An important element in childhood obesity is a dietary intervention. On the basis of experience and research, Epstein and Wing [47] suggest dividing food products into three categories: eating at one's heart content (green), eating moderately (orange) and forbidden to eat (red). This programme has the disadvantage that the emphasis is still laid on food restriction, which may lead to undesired side effects in children. Other programmes are more in favor of making the children follow the guidelines as prescribed by the National Institute for Food. In this approach, food is classified within a food pyramid, with, for example, eating varied and healthy food as a major principle. More attention is paid to what is still allowed, such as a lot of vegetables and fruit. These principles may go for the whole family and offer better guarantees for lifelong maintenance of the new eating habits [48].

In most obesity treatments, reduction of caloric intake is the most significant contribution to negative energy balance. Increased physical activity, however, also contributes to it, and may accelerate weight loss and improve maintenance of lost weight. Epstein and Wing [47] suggest initiating an exercise programme in which mainly aerobic exercises of moderate intensity are planned, such as cycling, swimming, walking, jogging, rope-skipping or rowing. These activities are planned in an exercise scheme, which stimulates children to take physical exercise for about 20 min a day.

The third important cornerstone is behavioral therapy. Interesting results are provided by Epstein et al. [49] who demonstrated the importance of behavioral techniques like self-monitoring, contracting, stimulus control and rewarding the child. The methods are discussed in the following paragraph. Most techniques can be seen as parts of a self-regulation training, as described by Harter [50] for children. Additionally, Graves et al. [51] investigated the positive effects including problem-solving. Finally, targeting the parents in a behavioral treatment of childhood obesity enhances the therapy results. In the treatment of Epstein and Wing [47], the child is only allowed the treatment if it has at least one obese parent and also if the parent is willing to follow a treatment programme. This, however, causes problems when the child or the parent loses weight, whereas the other party gains weight. Israel et al. [52] therefore chose to involve the parents in the treatment as assistant therapists. The parents are asked to continue at home what has been dealt with in the therapy and to help their child in the completion of the tasks. Our own experience is based on this latter approach. Golan et al. [53] describes a treatment for obese children in which solely the parents are involved. Now research is ongoing if this treatment is as effective in comparison with a family-based treatment.

Programmes incorporating dietary advices and physical activity programmes in a behavioral-therapeutic approach can realize 5–20% weight reduction [47, 54, 55]. A recently completed long-term follow-up study of children treated for obesity, conducted at the Ghent University, indicated that the children that had followed an educational behavioral-therapeutic group programme were still 17% below their initial overweight 4 years later (effect size: 1.07), whereas the group of children that received an advice only once, showed a 6% decrease of their initial overweight, or an effect size of 0.25 [56]. An overview of a protocol is described in table 1.These findings confirm Epstein's results and justify the use of an educational behavioral-therapeutic protocol in the treatment of obese children, with three components: healthy food, moderate daily exercises and behavioral techniques whereby the parents were actively involved in one way or another.

To conclude, family behavioral therapy has already produced positive results in controlled studies with maintenance of a long-term weight loss [44, 49, 55, 56].

Indications for the Treatment of Child Obesity

The Weight Criterion
In a clinical-medical research, the skinfold thickness is used to estimate the amount of body fat. This method, however, is liable to miscalculations: especially in case of severe obesity the skinfold thickness cannot be determined

Table 1. Protocol spread over 6 sessions

1	• diary tasks (nutrition and exercise) • instructions about nutrition and exercise • building a contract
2	• discussion of the tasks • looking for realistic modifications in eating and exercising habits • instructions about nutrition and exercise • new contract
3	• contract evaluation • looking for realistic modifications in eating and exercising habits • instructions about nutrition and exercise • new contract
4	• contract evaluation • looking for realistic modifications in eating and exercising habits • instructions about nutrition and exercise • stimulus control strategies • problem-solving (i) identification of difficult moments • new contract
5	• contract evaluation • further building new eating and exercise habits • behavioral exercise, modelling • problem-solving (i) identification of difficult moments • new contract
6	• problem-solving thinking (ii) discussion of difficult moments • role play, modelling

univocally. In adults, a BMI gives good estimates of the existing fat body mass and a BMI greater than 30 is considered as a criterion for obesity. However, this can only be used as absolute value for fully grown adolescents.

International guidelines for defining overweight and obesity in children and adolescents were recently published [57]. BMI standards were expressed as 'percentiles' for children and will become the 'golden standard' for determining the degree of obesity [57, 58]. Children and adolescents between the 85th and 95th percentiles of BMI have been described as being 'at risk for overweight', while children exceeding the 95th percentiles are described as 'at risk for obesity' [12]. An alternative method for defining obesity is to identify those BMI scores that would 'project' to a BMI of 25 (i.e. overweight) or 30 (i.e. obese) at 18 years of age. Using data from Brazil, Great Britain, Hong Kong, Netherlands, Singapore, and the United States, percentiles were available now for different age groups.

When trying to design the weight evolution of a particular child, overweight can also be expressed in terms of percentage of the current weight to the 'standard BMI', which is comparable with percentile of 50. A deviation of more than 20% is already considered as overweight. Child obesity represents a range of forms with on the one hand moderately obese children (20–40% overweight), obese children (40–60% overweight) and severely obese children (>60% overweight).

Example: A boy of 8 years weighs 43 kg and is 131 cm tall. The standard for a boy of this age and length is 26.4 kg. This is 16.6 kg too much. His BMI (weight/length^2 × 100) is 25 and, using the BMI standards for his age, a standard BMI (= percentile 50) is 15.8, so his overweight is, based on BMI standards, 58%. Percentile >95.

With respect to the indications for treatment, so far, no study is known demonstrating that obese girls suffer more or less than obese boys. It therefore seems highly recommendable to treat both.

Age

The age of the child also plays an important role in the indication for treatment. Research has demonstrated that, at the age of 10, approximately 80% of the obese children remain obese in the future [4]. It is generally assumed that from that age onwards intervention is absolutely necessary. Even better, based on the study of Whitaker et al. [4], and using an 'early intervention' perspective, obese children between the ages of 7 and 10 are indicated as ideal candidates for treatment. From the point of view of prevention, the group of 5- to 7-year-olds must be 'followed'. The chances of spontaneous recovery, however, are still great then. The following components appear to be important here: the weight of the parents, economic class and current eating habits [4].

Counterindications

There are a number of syndromes in which childhood obesity is merely a symptom of an underlying syndrome (e.g. Prader-Willi syndrome, endocrine disorders; see [14]). These syndromes are rare. Yet, parents are often convinced that there ought to be a medical 'cause' in their child. It is therefore advisable always to call in a doctor to exclude these syndromatic expressions of childhood obesity.

In some children underlying emotional problems have been observed, such as coping with a great loss or serious family problems. These children may profit from a weight loss programme, but this will never be enough. Here, a two-track policy is opted for, i.e. focussing on the weight problem and tackling the underlying problems at the same time. Furthermore, a more personal approach will be necessary when binge-eating episodes are already reported. An adequate screening in advance is therefore imperative. It can spare the child, the parents and the therapist the frustration of an unsuccessful therapy.

The treatment described below is a non-diet approach and no weight loss is aimed, only weight control. However, this is not suitable in its present form for children with very severe overweight (>80%). Furthermore, treatment in childhood profits from the fact that children are still growing and this growth requires energy. However, in fully grown adolescents this energy expenditure diminish and weight control will be much more difficult to install. Therefore, the programme described here especially appears to be a good choice for the treatment of children ageing between 7 and 12, with an overweight between 20 and 80%. Positive support and goodwill from the environment is advisable.

CBT Methods in the Treatment of Obese Children

Stimulus Control

For obese children it is helpful to have fewer supplies in the house and to store the necessary supplies in as few cupboards as possible. Furthermore it is recommended not to put the pots on the table and to throw the leftovers away immediately. Children are strongly advised to reduce the number of places where they eat to a minimum, preferably to only one place, for example the kitchen, even if there are crisps on Saturday evening. It is also recommended to do nothing else but eating during the meal and to avoid other activities such as reading, watching television or making telephone calls. Moreover, it is advisable to develop the habit of eating only at fixed hours. The National Institute for Food suggests the following scheme: breakfast between 7 and 8 a.m., a morning snack at 10, lunch between 12 and 13 p.m., an afternoon snack at 4, dinner around 6 p.m. and if so desired a final snack at 8 o'clock in the evening. Researchers assume that as one eats in more situations, there are more and more environmental stimuli reminding of food, whereas reducing these situations extinguishes the reminding value of an environmental stimulus. This behavioral-therapeutic technique appeared to be the first to be successful within the treatment for obesity.

Diaries

The diary is an important tool in the treatment of obese children in order to learn self-regulation skills. Everything a child eats and drinks and how much, is daily written down in the diary. The child preferably keeps the diary itself, at school as well. As for younger children, the mother can help. The child may then be involved in the task by for example coloring a green or a red ball each time he/she eats or by sticking the packing of a healthy snack in the diary. This diary is very useful to get an idea of the daily eating habits of the child. If persistent bad eating habits are involved, it is recommended to write down all situations that provoke these habits. Already at the beginning of the treatment, a second diary is introduced in an identical way: the exercise diary. In this diary the child writes down all forms of exercise it takes in the course of a week.

Contracts

Self-regulation implicates that realistic goals are formulated, together with the child. Once a week preferably one food-related and one exercise-related issue deserving special attention and this is worked out together with the child, which leads to an agreement in the form of a contract. On the contract there are clear, realistic tasks, such as drinking water at meals, as well as univocal evaluation criteria, such as '5 of 7 days'. The objective is that the child, with a little effort, succeeds in achieving the objective it has set in advance. Consequently, this objective is different for each child, which requires a personal approach.

A lot of children enjoy receiving a small material when the contract is evaluated. We recommend to chose rewards appropriate to the treatment, such as a ball, a skipping-rope, a cassette with dance music, or saving for a social activity every week, such as playing a party game together, dancing during the session, etc. The child can be stimulated to make a list of gifts wanted.

The contract evaluation is an important learning moment for the child. It is recommendable to always follow the rules for 'good feedback'. This means that social reinforcement in the form of encouragement and compliments for what went well is still essential. In doing so, the child himself should particularly look at what goes well already. The child is thus given the chance to experience small successes, which increases the chance to develop self-regulation.

Self-Evaluation and Self-Reinforcement

Children must learn to evaluate themselves positively with an open mind, preferably on the basis of the contract, and to encourage themselves for what went well, such as: 'well done', 'that's the way!', 'I'm doing well'. If a child fails to follow the contract, or only partially, it must learn to adjust itself, for example: 'I had a good start this week, next week I'll do better' or 'I'm already quite successful in eating vegetables, but at 4 o'clock I still have a difficult time not eating sweets'.

Problem-Solving Thinking

When reading the diaries, it will soon become clear that obese children often have to cope with difficult situations. Examples: What do you do when you're at home alone and feel like eating? What do you do on a birthday party when offered sweets? What if granny wishes to spoil you? What do you do with your pocket money? As it is gradually becoming a common procedure in several cognitive behavioral-therapeutic interventions with children, the children are taught coping and problem-solving skills. The child learns how to analyze a difficult situation, to think of and to evaluate several solutions. In searching different alternative solutions for 'difficult moments with respect to eating', the following rules of thumb can be useful: (1) avoid the situation; (2) do something else in that situation; (3) participate in the situation, but to a lesser extent, and (4) participate and do a physical exercise afterwards.

Behavior Training and Homework Tasks

During the sessions it is preferable to regularly train new forms of eating behavior. Each good behavior modification can only be established if practiced a lot. Examples are: to eat slowly, to chew properly, to avoid reading while eating, to wait for a moment before deciding on a second helping, to taste nothing in advance, to avoid lingering at the table. Also tasting unknown food products (vegetables, fruit) or experimenting with new healthy preparations may be on this list. Furthermore, new exercises are done as well, such as rope-skipping, abdominal exercises, learning a dance. Next, the children are asked to practice what they have learned further at home. The homework task is written down on the contract.

At a later stage in the therapy, the problem-solving alternatives are practiced as well, often in the form of a role play. This allows an obese child to learn to say 'No' when it is presented something sweet. If a child is being pestered, it can also learn skills to react with dignity. It is also possible that new skills are taught to learn to cope with moments of stress, boredom or distress (e.g. relaxation training).

Group Pressure and a Model Attitude of the Therapist

The treatment described here is preferably given in a small group. Group sessions are experienced as being more pleasant, but have the additional advantage that children can learn a lot from each other. This technique is defined as observational learning or modelling. The therapist can even stimulate observational learning by constantly acting as a model himself. In doing so, he can apply the 'thinking aloud' technique, which will mainly enhance the self-regulation and the problem-solving thinking. The children may also encourage each other and even put pressure on each other. Certain rewards may then be kept in the form of for example a group thermometer. Research has demonstrated that this form of treatment is preferable [55, 56]. Working with groups may also help keeping down the treatment costs. Moreover, people are more inclined to follow a treatment protocol.

Psychoeducation

Time and again the children appear to have practically no idea about the development of overweight and what is the best thing to do then. This can be visually explained to children by means of pictures, such as a pair of scales. It is also necessary to explain the difference between fats, carbohydrates and proteins, and what exactly happens with these elements in the body. Sometimes this may look like a lesson in biology. Here, a multidisciplinary team, were a dietician can contribute and discuss the diaries is recommended. When discussing the diaries, the therapist should be well informed about the directions to maintain a stable intake-expenditure balance, as prescribed by the National Institute for Food. Sometimes simple advices will do, such as 'to drink water' at meals; to choose low-fat products, to eat a carrot when you're hungry in between meals, to take breakfast, etc. Research has demonstrated that the chances of weight recovery are already good if motivated families are well informed, if some basic principles are explained to them in one or a few sessions and if they are given a clear manual.

Booster Sessions

In the treatment of obesity it is more and more assumed that a long-term follow-up is imperative [7]. Sustaining the new lifestyle remains quite a task. Studies indicate that the organization of control sessions after treatment, so-called booster sessions, is the most advisable technique to assure long-term behavior modification. The booster sessions can for example be organized every month, even one or two years after treatment. Booster sessions can be organized individually, but with children they are more often organized in the form of family conversations. In such sessions a problem-solving strategy is used, mainly looking for possibilities for the implementation of the previously learned issues in the living environment of the child. There is the suspicion that booster sessions prevent extinction of the newly learned eating habits, but it further appears that these sessions are mainly useful when self-regulation threatens to fail or when people have a setback (for example when they've gained a few pounds). For that purpose, 'techniques for the prevention of relapse' have been developed. These have been designed to support the patient when he for one reason or another threatens to abandon the programme, since, after a setback, the child runs the risk of losing courage, or having the reaction 'I've had enough' and does not find the motivation necessary to go on. In this way agreements can be made such as 'a bad day is not a bad programme', or 'today is a bad day, but tomorrow I'll start a new', or 'also mountaineers sometimes have to descend a little to be able to climb again with renewed courage'.

Dealing with Resistance

Research bears evidence that people are more inclined to be opposed to change if they have the feeling that this change is imposed or if they anyhow do not experience any freedom of making their own choice in this matter. Already at the outset of a treatment it is therefore advisable to investigate whether the obese child wishes to be treated and whether it has enough reasons of its own to go into treatment. In some cases it may be necessary to compare the pros and contras of a treatment versus the pros and contras of no treatment at all. Furthermore, there is evidence that the child is preferably left some freedom to plan its meals, snacks and physical activities. The more a child has the feeling that it can decide for itself, the more it will feel involved in the treatment and the smaller the chance of resistance. In this respect, for example, a list of healthy snacks may be drawn up, having the child decide for itself which snack it will take on the next day. It is also highly recommended to keep the favorite dishes on the menu, but to dose them, and to keep a complete freedom of choice for particular food areas (e.g. vegetables and fruit). Anyhow, it is not advisable to consider certain unhealthy snacks as 'absolutely forbidden' products: that which is forbidden will become very attractive, which will increase the attractiveness of the product as well as the chance to taste it secretly.

Role Played by the Parents and the Family

The other family members and first and foremost the parents of the obese child can be very supportive. However, there are different ways to involve parents in the treatment. In our approach, at the end of each session, one parent (or both parents) is invited to go through the contract together with the therapist. In doing so, it is examined whether the goals of the contract can be implemented,

Braet

i.e. whether the house can be organized so that the child is not constantly stimulated to eat and whether they can put healthy rather than unhealthy purchases on the shopping list. They are further encouraged to cycle together with their child, to plan a walk on Sundays or to try out a new healthy recipe. The influence of the environment is thus more indirect and in function of the patient.

On the other hand, this method also offers the possibility of helping the parents in adjusting their (parental) approach with respect to their child. They learn how to set clear and realistic rules, how to be consistent, how to watch the contracts and to give good feedback to their child. This often restores peace and quiet in the family, since there are fewer conflicts about when they should eat, and about what should be/should not be eaten. So, they are no longer discussions and doubts about how to realize a weight control program. If a child cannot live up to its contract, the parents do not have to blame the child for this, but they can write it down in the child's diary. The contract is then evaluated during the session under mediation of the therapist. If they are faced with problems, the parents can also learn problem-solving thinking. This is for example necessary if other family members or the grandparents are not willing to give up old habits or if the parents fail to provide the child with healthy alternatives. In that case, a more personal treatment may be necessary, which may lead to separate talks with the parents besides the treatment of the obese child. The contacts with the parents are often more difficult than the contacts with the child and require a specialized behavioral-therapeutic approach. It is advisable to take a non-accusatory, empathizing attitude here, and to look for possible solutions for the existing problems in a cooperative atmosphere. In many cases the therapist will demonstrate the suggested advices and feedback procedures in the session.

As described above, the parents of these children often find it difficult to set clear limits and to make concrete arrangements with their child. In such cases, the treatment for overweight necessarily implies acting on the parenting skills, as described by Patterson [59]. Important parenting skills can be learned: positive parental behavior, rule setting, disciplining, avoiding harsh punishment and inconsistent disciplining, and increasing appropriate rewarding. A pilot study revealed hopeful prospects for this approach [Moens and Braet, unpubl. data].

If problems arise in the parent-child interaction, it may be useful to also examine the thoughts and convictions of the parents. It could be recommendable to discuss their cognitions and thoughts about their child, their beliefs in the program they had to follow and about their attributions on the causes of childhood obesity. Cognitive therapy has shown that daily patterns of thought are guided by people's convictions and that these patterns of thought will determine the way of thinking of parents as well as their feelings and behavior.

The convictions may amongst others relate to 'I want to be a good mother' or 'I don't want to fail' and 'I want to see my child happy'. Specific cognitive techniques are used to make these convictions more explicit, to adjust or to modify them.

Some parents are very busy and give up early. Others are but little informed about good eating habits, whereas yet other parents report family conflicts. In some cases cooperation with other experts is possible. Information about good eating habits can be given by means of leaflets or cooking evenings and is preferably organized with the help of a dietician. In case there are family conflicts, a family therapist or a couple therapist can be called in. Further research will have to determine the number of families that need additional guidance. In case a family or a child threatens to drop out, the therapists have the possibility to contact the family themselves and, together with them, to examine whether the usually practical obstacles that hinder them can as yet be eliminated. Even when the parents report not being able to cooperate, the child cannot be deprived of its right to treatment for obesity.

Open Questions of Childhood Obesity Research: Future Prospects

There is considerable inter-individual variation in response to interventions such that not all children maintain weight loss. Follow-up research indicates that only 1 of 3 obese children reaches a weight that is beneath 20% [49, 56]. So, most of the children will remain overweight for the rest of their lives. Moreover, approximately 15% of the children keep gaining weight. This number increases up to 30% when the long-term evolutions are included [56]. Although research has shown that longer obesity treatment is associated with larger weight losses in adults, no research has examined how the length of treatment influences outcome in obese children [46].

Further research will probably reveal the underlying causes and whether interview indicators will be found already during the intake that are good predictors of a negative therapy outcome. One research showed that the assumed parameters such as the presence of emotional eating, external eating, dietary eating or the presence of psychopathology are not withheld in a regression analysis with weight loss as measure for therapy success. The only predictor of a long-term favorable outcome is initial weight loss, measured 3 months after the intake [55]. Furthermore, research bears evidence that the degree of success in the first year is predictive of the success 5 years after treatment [56].

Research on childhood obesity must teach us to better select the appropriate treatments for the appropriate children. As Jelalian and Saelens [44] noted,

'Much of the adolescent treatment research lacks methodological rigor, or fails to demonstrate short- or long-term success. There is much to be gained from examining how to adapt successful adult and/or child obesity programs for adolescents.' Also, for those fitting a specific genetic profile or for those who fail to respond to behavioral treatment, new interventions need to be considered. Further advances may lead to – although disputable – pharmacological interventions, surgery or inpatient treatment [60].

The most successful programs are those that incorporate a multidimensional approach characterized by the inclusion of diet, exercise and the application of behavior modification principles. However, few studies have compared the effects of one approach, while holding other aspects of the treatment constant. For example, although the results of studies including parents in a family based approach are very encouraging, there are many unanswered questions about how parental influences can enhance treatment effects [46]. We still do not know what the working ingredients are. Research is needed in understanding the best dietary, physical activity, and behavior change approaches to maximize treatment effects [46]. Sometimes a standard CBT-treatment is not advised, but a more personal approach. The decision to start a personal guidance programme should become clear during the intake procedure. This means that the multidisciplinary team tries to assess to what extent the current parent-child relationship will allow application of techniques and whether there are some indications yet for interfering with behavioral problems in the child. For motivated families that manage on their own to establish a healthy way of life and to stabilize the weight of their child, a few dietary advices will be enough to carry on, and psychological guidance will not be necessary. Given the diversity of health complications associated with obesity, intervention studies might expand outcome measures to include indexes of fitness, blood pressure, lipids, other heath-related variables, as well as psychological well-being or interpersonal functioning. Including such measures would provide a fuller picture of the overall effectiveness of behavioral interventions.

The goals for treating childhood obesity are regulating body weight. Although the treatment described here aimed at weight management, the psychologist will also have to pay attention to the psychological sequelae of obesity. He should give the child time to tell about the harassments or about its feelings of guilt and shame. Furthermore, the therapist should help the child learn to accept that it has a weight problem. In many cases, the behavioral therapist should mainly support the child. To this end the psychologist can do exercises that enhance the self-image of the child [61]. Therefore, it is also the goal of the treatment that the child will continue to enjoy eating without gaining weight and that it will moreover become proud of being able to control its weight.

The obese child and its parents should know full well that the tasks should be carried out further after treatment as well. Obese children will have to pay attention to their predisposition throughout their lives [14]. The current environment is arguably conducive for weight regain among obese children attempting to maintain weight loss. More research is planned to investigate whether weight regain can be prevented if the treatment is followed by individualized booster sessions in which the children learn maintenance strategies or relapse prevention techniques. Recently, Latner et al. [62] already argued that continuous care of indefinite duration may be necessary to achieve long-term treatment effects in most obese people. Furthermore, compliance to the treatment is another issue of concern. More studies are needed which focus on children who dropped out of treatment and why they do so. Nor do we know what the mediators of treatment change are. One solution may be studies that focus more on the documentation of the mechanisms of change and less on the weight change itself.

A question that is now under discussion is the generalizability of the treatment principles discussed here. In the 'Clinical Handbook of Psychological Disorders' Brownell and O'Neil [63] describe a recent treatment protocol for obese adults. There is great similarity with the programmes for children: the goal is no longer weight loss, but lifestyle modification. In doing so, both poles of the energy balance are targeted through education and cognitive behavioral-therapeutic techniques. This change of view on obesity treatment in adults has recently been outlined by Cooper et al. [64] and includes new ideas primarily on overcoming the problem of posttreatment weight regain. However, whether other techniques, useful in adult treatment, like cognitive strategies, will be easy to implement in childhood obesity, remains to be seen [65]. Although progress has been made in treating obesity in childhood, new developments are needed to improve long-term weight regulation.

Conclusions

Biological and psychological models to explain for the onset of child obesity are described. Medical as well as psychological and psychosocial consequences are discussed afterwards. Next, therapy indications, like weight criterion and age of the child are proposed. In order to tackle the problem of obesity in children, approaches are needed that succeeded in installing a balance between energy intake end energy expenditure. Evidence-based programmes are summarized. It is stated that teaching children to manage their energy balance by performing more physical activities and by changing their eating styles give more prospects than going on a diet. Strong emphasis is put on the therapeutic goal: self-regulation of a healthy lifestyle. This is achieved through behavioral techniques. The methods are discussed. Finally, problems and open questions of childhood obesity research are presented. Although weight control programs are hopeful with respect to their goals of 'weight control' and preventing further weight gain, follow-up research will be presented that indicated that most of the children will still have moderate overweight for the rest of their lives.

References

1 Fredriks AM, van Buuren S, Wit JM, Verloove-Vanhorick SP: Body index measurements in 1996–7 compared with 1980. Arch Dis Child 2000;82:107–112.
2 Flegal KM, Troiano RP: Changes in the distribution of body mass index of adults and children in the US population. Int J Obes Relat Metab Disord 2000;24:807–818.
3 Dietz WH: Health consequences of obesity in youth: Childhood predictors of adult disease. Pediatrics 1998;101:518–525.
4 Whitaker RC, Wright JA, Pepe MS, Seidel KD, Dietz WH: Predicting obesity in young adulthood from childhood and parental obesity. N Engl J Med 1997;337:869–873.
5 Mossberg HO: 40-year follow-up of overweight children. Lancet 1989;ii:491–493.
6 Freedman DS, Dietz WH, Srinivasan SR, Berenson GS: The relation of overweight to cardiovascular risk factors among children and adolescents: The Bogalusa Heart Study. Pediatrics 1999; 103:1175–1182.
7 Wilson GT: Behavioral treatment of childhood obesity: Theoretical and practical implications. Health Psychol 1994;13:371–372.
8 Garner DM, Wooley SC: Confronting the failure of behavioral and dietary treatments for obesity. Clin Psychol Rev 1991;11:729–780.
9 Bouchard C, Pérusse L, Rice T, Rao DC: The genetics of human obesity; in Bray G, Bouchard C, James PT (eds): Handbook of Obesity. New York, Marcel Dekker, 1998, pp 157–190.
10 Dietz WH, Gortmaker SL: Do we fatten our children at the television set? Obesity and television viewing in children and adolescents. Pediatrics 1985;75:807–812.
11 Sallis JF, Broyles SL, Frank-Spohrer G, Berry CC, Davis TB, Nader PR: Child's home environment in relation to the mother's adiposity. Int J Obes Relat Metab Disord 1995;19:190–197.
12 Berkowitz RI, Stunkard AJ: Development of childhood obesity; in Wadden AW, Stunkard AJ (eds): Handbook of Obesity Treatment. New York, Guilford Press, 2002.
13 Bouchard C, Tremblay A, Despres JP, Nadeau A, Lupien PJ, Theriault G, Dussault J, Moorjani S, Pinault S, Fournier G: The response to long-term overfeeding in identical twins. N Engl J Med 1990;322:1477–1482.
14 Bouchard C: Genetic influences on body weight and shape; in Brownell KD, Fairburn CG (eds): Eating Disorders and Obesity: A Comprehensive Handbook. New York, Guilford Press, 1995, pp 21–26.
15 Schachter S, Rodin J: Obese Humans and Rats. Washington, Erlbaum/Halsted, 1974.
16 Rodin J, Slochower J: Externality in the nonobese: Effects of environmental responsiveness on weight. J Pers Soc Psychol 1976;33:338–344.
17 Schlundt DG, Taylor D, Hill JO, Sbrocco T, Pope-Cordle J, Kasser T, Arnold D: A behavioral taxonomy of obese female participants in a weight-loss program. Am J Clin Nutr 1991;53: 1151–1158.
18 Goodman E, Whitaker RC: A prospective study of the role of depression in the development and persistence of adolescent obesity. Pediatrics 2002;110:497–504.
19 Braet C, Van Strien T: Assessment of emotional, externally induced and restrained eating behaviour in nine to twelve-year-old obese and non-obese children. Behav Res Ther 1997;35:863–873.
20 Pine DS, Cohen P, Brook J, Coplan JD: Psychiatric symptoms in adolescence as predictors of obesity in early adulthood: A longitudinal study. Am J Publ Hlth 1997;87:1303–1310.

21 Herman CP, Polivy J: Restrained eating; in Stunkard AJ (ed): Obesity. Philadelphia, Saunders, 1980, pp 208–225.

22 Jansen A: Bulimia nervosa effectief behandelen. Een handleiding voor therapeuten. Lisse, Swets & Zeitlinger, 1993.

23 Fairburn CG, Welch SL, Doll HA, Davies BA, O'Connor ME: Risk factors for bulimia nervosa: A community-based case-control study. Arch Gen Psychiatry 1997;54:509–517.

24 Decaluwe V, Braet C: Prevalence of binge-eating disorder in obese children and adolescents seeking weight-loss treatment. Int J Obes Rel Metab Dis 2003;27:404–409.

25 Birch LL: The acquisition of food acceptance patterns in children; in Boakes RA, Pooplewell DA, Burton LR (eds): Eating Habits. Food, Physiology and Learned Behaviour, vol V. New York, Wiley, 1987, pp 107–131.

26 Johnson SL, Birch LL: Parents' and children's adiposity and eating style. Pediatrics 1994;94: 653–661.

27 Drucker RR, Hammer LD, Agras WS, Bryson S: Can mothers influence their child's eating behavior? J Dev Behavl Pediatr 1999;20:88–92.

28 Laessle RG, Uhl H, Lindel B, Muller A: Parental influences on laboratory eating behavior in obese and non-obese children. International journal of obesity and related metabolic disorders. J Int Assoc Study Obesity 2001;25(suppl 1):S60–S62.

29 Strauss CC, Smith K, Frame C, Forehand R: Personal and interpersonal characteristics associated with childhood obesity. J Pediatr Psychol 1985;10:337–343.

30 Bray G: Effects of obesity on health and happiness; in Brownell KD, Foreyt JP (eds): Handbook of Eating Disorders: Physiology, Psychology, and Treatment of Obesity. New York, Basic Books, 1986.

31 Rodin M, Price J, Sanchez F, McElligot S: Derogation, exclusion, and unfair treatment of persons with social flaws: Controllability of stigma and the attribution of prejudice. Pers Soc Psychol Bull 1989;15:439–451.

32 Braet C, Mervielde I, Vandereycken W: Psychological aspects of childhood obesity: A controlled study in a clinical and nonclinical sample. J Pediatr Psychol 1997;22:59–71.

33 Kimm SY, Sweeney CG, Janosky JE, MacMillan JP: Self-concept measures and childhood obesity: A descriptive analysis. J Dev Behav Pediatr 1991;12:19–24.

34 Stradmeijer M, Bosch J, Koops W, Seidell J: Family functioning and psychosocial adjustment in overweight youngsters. Int J Eating Disord 2000;27:110–114.

35 Friedman MA, Brownell KD: Psychological correlates of obesity: Moving to the next research generation. Psychol Bull 1995;117:3–20.

36 French SA, Perry CL, Leon GR, Fulkerson JA: Self-esteem and change in body mass index over 3 years in a cohort of adolescents. Obes Res 1996;4:27–33.

37 Epstein LH, Myers MD, Anderson K: The association of maternal psychopathology and family socioeconomic status with psychological problems in obese children. Obes Res 1996;4:65–74.

38 Banis HT, Varni JW, Wallander JL, Korsch BM, Jay SM, Adler R, Garcia-Temple E, Negrete V: Psychological and social adjustment of obese children and their families. Child Care Hlth Dev 1988;14:157–173.

39 Rössner S: Childhood obesity and adult consequences. Acta Paediatr 1998;87:1–5.

40 Gortmaker SL, Must A, Perrin JM, Sobol AM, Dietz WH: Social and economic consequences of overweight in adolescence and young adulthood. N Engl J Med 1993;329:1008–1012.

41 Stunkard AJ, Sobal J: Psychosocial consequences of obesity; in Fairburn CG, Brownell KD (eds): Eating Disorders and Obesity. A Comprehensive Handbook. New York, Guilford Press, 1995, pp 417–421.

42 Berkowitz R, Stunkard AJ, Stallings VA: Binge-eating disorder in obese adolescent girls. Ann NY Acad Sci 1993;699:200–206.

43 Decaluwe V, Braet C: Prevalence of binge-eating disorder in obese children and adolescents seeking weight-loss treatment. Int J Obes Rel Metab Disord 2003;27:404–409.

44 Jelalian E, Saelens BE: Empirically supported treatments in pediatric psychology: Pediatric obesity. J Pediatr Psychol 1999;24:223–248.

45 Epstein LH, Myers MD, Raynor HA, Saelens BE: Treatment of pediatric obesity. Pediatrics 1998; 101:554–570.

46   Goldfield GS, Raynor HA, Epstein LH: Treatment of pediatric obesity; in Wadden TA, Stunkard AJ (eds): Handbook of Obesity Treatment. New York, Guilford Press, 2002, pp 301–315.

47   Epstein LH, Wing RR: Behavioral treatment of childhood obesity. Psychol Bull 1987;101(3): 331–342.

48   Braet C: Treatment of obese children: A new rationale. Clin Child Psychol Psychiatry 1999;4: 579–591.

49   Epstein LH, Valoski A, Wing RR, McCurley J: Ten-year outcomes of behavioral family-based treatment for childhood obesity. Health Psychol 1994;13:373–383.

50   Harter S: A developmental perspective on some parameters of self-regulation in children; in Karoly P, Kanfer FH (eds): Self-Management and Behavior Change. New York, Pergamon, 1982, pp 165–204.

51   Graves T, Meyers AW, Clark L: An evaluation of parental problem-solving training in the behavioral treatment of childhood obesity. J Consult Clin Psychol 1988;56:246–250.

52   Israel AC, Stolmaker L, Sharp JP, Silverman WK, Simon LG: An evaluation of two methods of parental involvement in treating obese children. Behav Ther 1984;15:266–272.

53   Golan M, Fainaru M, Weizman A: Role of behaviour modification in the treatment of childhood obesity with the parents as the exclusive agents of change. Int J Obes Relat Metab Disord 1998; 22:1217–1224.

54   Braet C: Dikke Kinderen. Leuven/Amersfoort, Acco, 1995.

55   Braet C, Van Winckel M, Van Leeuwen K: Follow-up results of different treatment programs for obese children. Acta Paediatr 1997;86:397–402.

56   Braet C, Van Winckel M: Long-term follow-up of a cognitive behavioral treatment program for obese children. Behav Ther 2000;31:55–74.

57   Cole TJ, Bellizzi MC, Flegal KM, Dietz WH: Establishing a standard definition for child overweight and obesity worldwide: International survey. Br Med J 2000;320:1240–1243.

58   Rolland-Cachera MF, Cole TJ, Sempe M, Tichet J, Rossignol C, Charraud A: Body Mass Index variations: Centiles from birth to 87 years. Eur J Clinical Nutr 1991;45:13–21.

59   Patterson GR: Coercive Family Process. Eugene, Castalia Press, 1982.

60   Braet C, Tanghe A, Decaluwe V, Moens E, Rosseel Y: Inpatient treatment of children with obesity: Weight loss, psychosocial well being, and eating behavior. J Pediatr Psychol 2004;29:519–529.

61   Braet C: Action techniques for boosting self-esteem in obese children; in Verhofstadt-Denève L (ed): A Theoretical and Practical Guide to Action and Drama Techniques. London, Jessica Kingsley Publishers, 2000, pp 233–254.

62   Latner JD, Stunkard AJ, Wilson GT, Jackson ML, Zelitch DS, Labouvie E: Effective long-term treatment of obesity: A continuing care model. Int J Obesity Rel Metab Disord 2000;24:893–898.

63   Brownell KD, O'Neil PM: Obesity; in Barlow DH (ed): Clinical Handbook of Psychological Disorders. New York, Guilford Press, 1993, pp 318–361.

64   Cooper Z, Fairburn CG, Hawker DM (eds): Cognitive-Behavioral Treatment of Obesity: A Clinician's Guide. New York, Guilford Press, 2003.

65   Duffy G, Spence SH: The effectiveness of cognitive self-management as an adjunct to a behavioural intervention for childhood obesity: A research note. J Child Psychol Psychiatry 1993;34: 1043–1050.

Prof. Dr. C. Braet
Ghent University, Department of Developmental
Personality and Social Psychology, H. Dunantlaan 2
BE–9000 Ghent (Belgium)
Tel. +32 9 264 64 16, Fax +32 9 264 64 99, E-Mail Caroline.Braet@ugent.be

Munsch S, Beglinger C (eds): Obesity and Binge Eating Disorder.
Bibl Psychiatr. Basel, Karger, 2005, No 171, pp 138–148

· ·

Binge Eating Disorder: A New Eating Disorder or an Epiphenomenon of Obesity?

Brunna Tuschen-Caffier, Claudia Schlüssel

Department of Psychology, University of Bielefeld,
Bielefeld, Germany

Binge eating disorder (BED) has been included in Appendix B of the *Diagnostic and Statistical Manual of Mental Disorders* (ed 4, DSM-IV) [1] as a disorder with research criteria requiring further study. The following criteria have to be fulfilled to provisionally diagnose BED:

- Recurrent episodes of binge eating which means eating definitely more than other people would eat under similar circumstances. Additionally, a sense of lack of control during binge-eating episodes has to be diagnosed.
- Binge-eating episodes are associated at least with three typical features like eating much more rapidly than normal, eating until feeling uncomfortably full, eating large amounts of food when not feeling physically hungry.
- Patients feel distressed regarding binge eating.
- Binge eating occurs at least during 2 days a week for a period of at least 6 months.
- Binge eating is not associated with inappropriate compensatory behaviors (e.g. purging).

The introduction of the BED diagnosis within DSM-IV has stimulated a lot of research over the past decade as well as many critical questions concerning the utility of this new diagnosis. One question is whether individuals with BED differ from individuals who are just obese. Another question is whether BED is a distinct new diagnosis or just a subtype of bulimia nervosa. The following chapter will present evidence-based arguments for the following claims: (a) BED is a clinical disorder; (b) BED is different from bulimia nervosa; (c) BED is different from non-BED obesity. Before we will argue for these claims, we will present epidemiological data on BED to show that BED is a widespread clinical phenomenon.

Epidemiology of BED

Epidemiological research plays an important role in answering the question if BED is distinct from other diagnostic categories for eating disorders.

Methodological Limitation. It is important to note that epidemiologic studies of BED are limited in methodology regarding the selection of populations and identification of cases [2]. At present, the most accepted method is the two-stage screening approach [3]. One limitation of this procedure is the poor response rate. Record-based studies, however, characterize only a minority of all cases whereas samples of special populations (e.g. social work students, high school girls) lack in their generalization to the general population.

One important source of measurement error is the wide range concerning the meaning of binge eating when used by the general public. Assessing self-report questionnaires leads to greater methodological limitations than interview-based assessment. The reason for this is that in the latter the term binge eating can be more clarified. Therefore, for example, prevalence rates based on self-reports tend to be higher then those on interview-based methods [4, 5].

Not only do assessment strategies influence prevalence results, but furthermore, prevalence rates differ depending on the sample chosen (e.g. community sample, students, inpatients).

Another example illustrates how prevalence rates differ in relation to criteria used to determine BED. Hay [6] found a prevalence rate of 1% for BED using the DSM-IV frequency criteria for binge eating [1] whereas a prevalence of 2.5% was estimated using the broader Oxford criteria by Fairburn and Cooper [7].

This methodological limitation should be taken into mind when reading the following epidemiological results.

Prevalence of BED
Prevalence comprises the total number of cases in the population and indicates the demand for care. A short review of prevalence rates for BED is illustrated in table 1.

The prevalence rates in community-based studies vary from 0.7% [8, 26] to 2.5% [21], and, respectively, 3.3% [14] for the general female Austrian population. A prevalence range from 0.28% [9] to 5.3% [21] was estimated in

Table 1. Prevalence rates for BED

Reference	Sample		Assessment	Prevalence rate	
				female	male
Basdevant et al. [8]	community sample and patient samples	France	self-report questionnaires	0.7% (community sample) 8.9% (private practice); 15.2% (hospital)	–
Cotrufo et al. [9]	group of 13- to 19-year-old females	Italy	two-stage procedure	0.28%	–
Diez-Quevedo et al. [10]	general hospital patients	Spain	PRIME-MD Patient Health Questionnaire (PHQ; Spitzer et al., 1994)	5.3 %	–
Ghaderi and Scott [11]	females age 18–30 years	Sweden	questionnaires	1.2%	–
Götestam and Agras [12]	community-based sample	Norway	self-report questionnaire	1.5% 3.2% (lifetime prev.)	–
Hay [6]	community-based sample	Australia	EDE	1%*–2.5%**	–
Kalman et al. [13]	outpatients weight management and nutritional counselling program		questionnaire and interview	22.2%	–
Kinzl et al. [14]	general female population	Austria	telephone interview	3.3%	
Kinzl et al. [15]	general male population	Austria	telephone interview	–	0.8%
Ramacciotti et al. [16]	obese people in treatment	Italy	Binge Eating Disorder Clinical Interview (BEDCI) [21]	12.1% (6-month prev.) 18.1% (lifetime prev.)	–
Ricca et al. [17]	overweight people in obesity treatments	Italy		7.5%	–

Study	Sample	Country	Assessment method	Prevalence	DSM-IV*/Oxford**
Robertson and Palmer [18]	women with a history of obesity		self-report measures and interview	1.5%	—
Smith et al. [19]			self-report instrument	1.5%	—
Spitzer at al. [20]	community-based sample	USA	self-report	2.5%	1.1%
Spitzer et al. [21]	college students	USA	self-report	2.8%	1.9%
	employees at medical centers	USA	self-report	5.3%	3.1%
	participants of weight control programs		self-report	29.7%	21.1%
Spitzer et al. [22]	primary care patients	USA	PRIME-MD Patient Health Questionnaire	6%	—
Spitzer et al. [23]	women recruited at obstetric-gynecology practices	USA	PRIME-MD Patient Health Questionnaire	4%	—
Striegel-Moore et al. [24]	NHLBI Growth and Health Study participants	USA	two-stage case finding method	2.7% (white women) 1.4 % (black women)	—
Thiels and Garthe [25]	social work students	Germany	Bulimic Investigatory Test Edinburgh (BITE; Henderson & Freeman, 1987)	3.8%	3.5%
Westenhöfer [26]	community-based sample	Germany	Interview and questionnaire	0.7%	0.7–1.5%

*DSM-IV frequency criteria for binge eating [1]. **Oxford criteria by Fairburn and Cooper [7].

studies focussing on special populations. The highest prevalence rates for BED were found in primary care or clinical samples, ranging from 4% [23] to 15.2% [8] and even up to 29.7% in samples consisting of participants in weight control programs [21].

Demographics

Concerning the demographics of subjects with BED most studies only focused on gender and ethnicity.

Gender. The majority of studies did not find gender differences comparing white women and white men on rates of BED. Nevertheless, men are less likely to meet the criteria for BED, although gender differences do not reach statistical significance (table 1). These findings, however, are preliminary because most studies of BED have only focused on female samples. According to Striegel-Moore and Cachelin [27], the gender imbalance concerning prevalence is less pronounced in BED then in other eating disorders. In reference to Lewingsohn et al. [28] men reported less distress over binge eating and used less extreme compensatory behavior then women.

Ethnicity. Most of the few studies on ethnic group differences are focused on blacks. Findings suggest that BED may be equal common among white and black women [29]. However, most of these findings were based on self-reports. Striegel-Moore et al. [24] reported that significantly more white women (2.7%) than black women (1.4%) met the criteria for BED (table 1). Pike et al. [30] examined eating disorder features and found significant differences between black and white women, e.g. black women with BED reported less concern about weight, shape and eating in relation to white women with BED. More research is needed in this field and an extension to other ethnic minority groups is necessary.

Taken together, epidemiological data show that BED is a widespread eating disturbance. But one of the questions is still whether this kind of eating disturbance is a distinct clinical disorder.

Claim 1: BED Is a Clinical Disorder

Preoccupation with body shape and weight has been considered to be a 'core' symptom of eating disorders [31]. Although body image disorder up until now has not been included in the DSM criteria for the diagnosis of BED several studies have shown that BED is quite comparable with bulimia nervosa (BN) and anorexia nervosa (AN) with respect to this symptom [32, 33]. Moreover, it has been shown that body image disturbances are more pronounced in obese binge eaters than in obese non-binge eaters [34, 35] as well as in slightly overweight BED subjects compared to controls [36]. For instance, Hilbert et al. [36] investigated psychological reactions to prolonged and repeated body image exposure in 30 female volunteers diagnosed with BED (DSM-IV) and 30 non-eating-disordered controls. In an experimental design, the participants of the study were exposed to their physical appearance in a mirror. The confrontation procedure was guided by a standardized interview manual and took place on two separate days. Self-reported mood, appearance self-esteem and frequency of negative cognitions were assessed repeatedly throughout the experiment. During body image exposure sessions, binge-eating disordered individuals showed significantly lower mood than controls while appearance self-esteem was diminished in both groups. Moreover, individuals diagnosed with BED consistently described themselves as fatter than non-eating-disordered individuals despite equivalent BMIs.

In line with these results it has been shown that weight and shape concerns of subjects with BED are comparable to those with bulimia nervosa and more pronounced than in obese non-bingeing controls [35, 37, 38]. Taking together the data indicate that BED is associated with marked body image distress.

Another similarity between BED and other eating disorders is that BED is associated with a high rate of past and present comorbidity with axis I and axis II disorders. For instance, Wilfley et al. [39] have analyzed comorbidity in 162 subjects with BED. One result of the study was that 33% of the subjects met at least one current comorbid axis I diagnosis. Most of the subjects (22%) were suffering from concurrent mood disorders. Concerning lifetime diagnosis 77% of the subjects met the criteria at least for one axis I disorder. Again, most of the lifetime diagnoses were on mood disorders (61%), especially major depression (58%). Additionally, many subjects met the criteria for at least one personality disorder (37%) and 14% met the criteria for more than one personality disorder. The most prevalent diagnoses were obsessive-compulsive personality disorder (14%), avoidant personality disorder (12%) and borderline personality disorder (9%).

Furthermore, in a population-based study of female twins it has been shown that obese women with binge eating reported about greater health dissatisfaction and higher rates of major medical disorders than obese non-bingeing women [40]. For instance, women with binge-eating reported about greater depression, anxiety, phobia and neurovegetative symptoms (e.g. agitation, insomnia, obsessive-compulsive traits) than just obese women.

Taken together, empirical studies have shown that BED is associated with severe clinical symptoms that allow to suppose that BED is a clinical disorder.

Claim 2: BED Is Different from Bulimia nervosa

To justify the utility of the new diagnostic category of BED it has to be shown that BED is a distinct eating disorder. Especially it has to be demonstrated that BED is different from bulimia nervosa. Up until now several studies indeed have shown that there are some differences between BED and BN, but these differences seem to be more quantitative than qualitative [41]. For instance, several laboratory studies have examined the eating behavior of patients with bulimia nervosa or with binge-eating disorder [42]. Although no single study has conducted a direct comparison, several studies used identical methods for the examination of the eating behavior of bulimics and BED subjects, thus allowing some preliminary comparisons between the eating behavior of these two eating disordered groups. Reviewing the literature, Walsh and Boudreau [42] noted three differences between BED and bulimics concerning their eating behavior in the lab: (a) The size of the average binge meal in the lab is greater in patients with bulimia nervosa than in patients with BED; (b) bulimics show a more disturbed pattern of food consumption during a binge meal than patients with BED; (c) during non-binge meals bulimics consume fewer calories than controls and far fewer calories than BED patients.

This indicates that the eating behavior of BED patients and bulimics – measured in the laboratory – is quite different although the DSM-IV criteria for binge eating are comparable for both groups. On the other hand, as Cooper and Fairburn [43] emphasized, distinguishing the eating behavior of BED patients from other forms of unstructured overeating is not quite easy, even if an investigator-based interview like the Eating Disorder Examination is used [7].

Considering the history of eating disorders, Striegel-Moore et al. [32] found that 150 BED subjects compared with 48 subjects with purging bulimia nervosa (BN) were less likely to have a history of anorexia nervosa and less likely to have been treated for an eating disorder. Moreover, as expected, subjects with BED were more often obese than subjects with purging or non-purging BN. On the other hand, Striegel-Moore et al. [32] did not find differences between subjects with BED and nonpurging BN (NP-BN) with respect to treatment history. This may be due to the small sample sizes of the NP-BN group (n = 14). Additionally, Hay and Fairburn [44] did not find significant differences between BED subjects and NP-BN regarding self-reported psychopathology, self-esteem or social adjustment. Concerning self-concept disturbances, moreover, in the study of Jacobi et al. [45], anorexic and bulimic patients as well as patients with BED displayed similar self-concept deficits.

Furthermore, Striegel-Moore et al. [32] did not find significant differences between BED and purging BN as well as non-purging BN according to weight and shape concern, or current or lifetime prevalence of nine major mental disorders.

Last but not least, if BED is a useful diagnostic category, clinicians should be able to prescribe a treatment that may be specific for the treatment of BED. Concerning this issue, Wilfley et al. [33] reviewed the literature and emphasized that overall research has shown that a variety of different psychological treatments appear to be comparably effective in reducing binge eating. For instance, cognitive-behavioral therapy (CBT) and interpersonal therapy (IPT) seem to produce highly similar results in the treatment of BED [46]. Concerning the treatment of bulimia nervosa, CBT seems to be the first-line treatment of choice [47]. For instance, comparing CBT wit IPT regarding the treatment of BN, at least at post-treatment CBT, was highly superior [48, 49].

Thus, taken together there is some evidence that BED and BN are different from each other (e.g. concerning the eating behavior, elevated rates of obesity, lower risk of anorexia nervosa in subjects with BED, responsiveness to CBT and alternative therapies). But up until now the claim that BED and BN are different disorders is somewhat tentative. Studies with lager sample sizes, especially according to NP-BN as well as prospective studies are needed to clarify whether BED is more similar to or different from BN, especially NP-BN.

Claim 3: BED Is Different from Non-BED Obesity

Several studies have shown that BED is associated with obesity [50–52]. However, it has also been found that obese individuals with BED differ from individuals who are just obese. For instance, several studies have found higher rates of psychiatric comorbidity in individuals with BED than in obese individuals without BED [53, 54]. Especially the rate of major depression was much higher in the obese BED group than in the non-BED obese; additionally, borderline personality disorder was much more prevalent in BED subjects than in the non-BED obese [54].

Moreover, BED subjects show a higher tendency to eat in response to emotional states and suffer from higher levels of eating psychopathology than non-BED obese subjects [33, 53, 54]. For instance, *body image distress* is considered as a core psychopathological feature of eating disorders and it has been found repeatedly that body image distress is more pronounced in obese BED subjects than in obese non-binge eaters [34, 35].

These findings indicate that BED is associated with much more impairment than obesity without BED. Taken together the results demonstrate that BED is not only an epiphenomenon of obesity but a distinctive subset of the obese population.

Conclusions

There is some evidence that the validity of BED as a diagnostic entity may be given. Subjects with BED are different from healthy controls in many aspects, e.g. overconcern with body weight and shape, comorbidity with axis I and axis II disorders or greater health dissatisfaction. Moreover, individuals with BED differ from those with other eating disorders like anorexia or bulimia nervosa (e.g. the eating behavior, the responsiveness to different psychological treatments). On the other hand, it has been difficult to distinguish BED from other forms of overeating, including NP-BN. Further research with larger sample sizes is needed to clarify whether BED for instance is really different from non-purging bulimia nervosa. Moreover, research should pay attention to refining the diagnostic criteria of BED as Cooper and Fairburn [43] already supposed. For instance, in our opinion body dissatisfaction should be added as a diagnostic criteria into the DSM-IV because there is evidence that subjects with BED show a pronounced overconcern with body weight and shape.

References

1   American Psychiatric Association: Diagnostic and Statistical Manual of Mental Disorders, ed 4, revised, 1994.
2   Hsu LKG: Epidemiology of the eating disorders. Psychiatr Clin N Am 1996;19:681–700.
3   Hoek HW, van Hoeken D: Review of the prevalence and incidence of eating disorders. Int J Eat Disord 2003;34:383–396.
4   Fairburn CG, Beglin SJ: Studies of the epidemiology of bulimia nervosa. Am J Psychiatry 1990;147:401–408.
5   Fairburn CG, Beglin SJ: Assessment of eating disorders: Interview or self-report questionnaire? Int J Eat Disord 1994;16:363–370.
6   Hay P: The epidemiology of eating disorder behaviors: An Australian community-based survey. Int J Eat Disord 1998;23:371–382.
7   Fairburn CG, Cooper Z: The eating disorder examination; in Fairburn CG, Wilson GT (eds): Binge Eating: Nature, Assessment, and Treatment, ed 12. New York, Guilford Press, 1993, pp 317–360.
8   Basdevant A, Pouillon M, Lahlou N, Le-Barzic M, Guy-Grand B: Prevalence of binge eating disorder in different populations of French women. Int J Eat Disord 1995;18:309–315.
9   Cortufo P, Barretta V, Monteleone P: An epidemiological study on eating disorders in two high schools in Naples. Eur Psychiatry 1997;12:342–344.
10 Diez-Quevedo C, Rangil T, Sanchez-Planell L, Kroenke K, Spitzer RL: Validation and utility of the patient health questionnaire in diagnosing mental disorders in 1003 general hospital Spanish inpatients. Psychosom Med 2001;63:679–686.
11 Ghaderi A, Scott B: Prevalence, incidence, and prospective risk factors for eating disorders. Acta Psychiatr Scand 2001;104:122–130.
12 Götestam KG, Agras WS: General population-based epidemiological study of eating disorders in Norway. Int J Eat Disord 1995;18:119–126.
13 Kalman D, Cascarano H, Krieger DR, Incledon T, Woolsey M: Frequency of binge eating disorder in an outpatient weight loss clinic. J Am Dietetic Assoc 2002;102:697–698.

14   Kinzl JF, Traweger C, Trefalt E, Mangweth B, Biebl W: Binge eating disorder in females: A population-based investigation. Int J Eat Dis 1999;25:287–292.

15   Kinzl JF, Traweger C, Trefalt E, Mangeweth B, Biebl W: Binge eating disorder in males: A population-based investigation. Eat Weight Disord 1999;4:169–174.

16   Ramacciotti CE, Coli E, Passaglia C, Lacorte M, Pea E, Dell'Osso L: Binge eating disorder: Prevalence and psychopathological features in a clinical sample of obese people in Italy. Psychiatry Res 2000;94:131–138.

17   Ricca V, Mannucci E, Moretti S, Di-Bernardo M, Zucchi T, Cabras PL, Rotella CM: Screening for binge eating disorder in obese outpatients. Compr Psychiatry 2000;41:111–115.

18   Robertson DN, Palmer RL: The prevalence and correlates of binge eating in a British community sample of women with a history of obesity. Int J Eat Disord 1997;22:323–327.

19   Smith DE, Marcus MD, Lewis CE, Fitzgibbon M, Schreiner P: Prevalence of binge eating disorder, obesity and depression in a biracial cohort of young adults. Ann Behav Med 1998;20: 227–232.

20   Spitzer RL, Devlin MJ, Walsh BT, Hasin D, Wing R, Marcus M, Stunkard A, Wadden T, Yanovski S, Agras S, Mitchell J, Nonas C: Binge eating disorder: A multisite field trial of the diagnostic criteria. Int J Eat Disord 1992;11:191–203.

21   Spitzer RL, Yanovski SZ, Wadden T, Wing R, Stunkard A, Devlin M, Mitschell J, Hasin D, Horne RL: Binge eating disorder: Its further validation in a multisided study. Int J Eat Disord 1993;13: 137–153.

22   Spitzer RL, Kroenke K, Williams JB: Validation and utility of a self-report version of PRIME-MD: The PHQ Primary Care Study. J Am Med Assoc 1999;282:1737–1744.

23   Spitzer RL, Williams JB, Kroenke K, Hornyak R, McMurray J: Validity and utility of the PRIME-MD patient health questionnaire in assessment of 3000 obstetric-gynecologic patients: The PRIME-MD Patient Health Questionnaire Obstetrics-Gynecology Study. Am J Obstet Gynecol 2000;183:759–769.

24   Striegel-Moore RH, Dohm FA, Kraemer HC, Taylor CB, Daniels S, Crawford PB, Schreiber GB: Eating disorders in white and black women. Am J Psychiatry 2003;106:1326–1331.

25   Thiels C, Garthe R: Prävalenz von Essstörungen unter Studierenden. Nervenarzt 2000;71: 552–558.

26   Westenhöfer J: Prevalence of eating disorders and weight control practices in Germany in 1990 and 1997. Int J Eat Disord 2001;29:477–481.

27   Striegel-Moore RH, Cachelin FM: Etiology of eating disorders in women. Couns Psychol 2001; 29:635–661.

28   Lewinsohn PM, Seeley JR, Moerk KC, Striegel-Moore RH: Gender differences in eating disorder symptoms in young adults. Int J Eat Disord 2002;32:426–440.

29   Striegel-Moore RH, Franko DL: Epidemiology of binge eating disorder. Int J Eat Disord 2003; 34:19–29.

30   Pike KM, Dohm FA, Striegel-Moore RH, Wilfley DE, Fairburn CG: A comparison of black and white women with binge eating disorder. Am J Psychiatry 2001;158:1455–1460.

31   Fairburn CG: Eating disorders; in Clark DM, Fairburn DG (eds): Science and Practice of Cognitive Behaviour Therapy. London, Oxford University Press, 1993, pp 209–241.

32   Striegel-Moore RH, Cachelin FM, Dohm FA, Pike KM, Wifley DE, Fairburn DG: Comparison of binge eating disorder and bulimia nervosa in a community sample. Int J Eat Disord 2001;29: 157–165.

33   Wilfley DE, Wilson GT, Agras WS: The clinical significance of binge eating disorder. Int J Eat Disord 2003;34:S96–S106.

34   Striegel-Moore RH, Wilson GT, Wilfley DE, Elder KA, Brownell KD: Binge eating in an obese community sample. Int J Eat Disord 1998;23:27–37.

35   Wilfley DE, Schwartz MB, Spurrell EB, Fairburn CG: Using the Eating Disorder Examination to identify the specific psychopathology of binge eating disorder. Int J Eat Disord 2000;27:259–269.

36   Hilbert A, Tuschen-Caffier B, Vögele C: Effects of prolonged and repeated body image exposure in binge eating disorder. J Psychosom Res 2002;52:137–144.

37   Kalarchian MA, Wilson GT, Brolin RE, Bradely L: Binge eating in bariatric surgery patients. Int J Eat Disord 1998;23:89–92.

38   Stunkard AJ, Allison KC: Binge Eating Disorder: Disorder or marker? Int J Eat Disord 2003;34:S107–S116.

39   Wilfley DE, Friedman MA, Dounchis JZ, Stein RI, Welch RR, Ball SA: Comorbid psychopathology in binge eating disorder: Relation to eating disorder severity at baseline and following treatment. J Consult Clin Psychol 2000;68:641–649.

40   Bulik CM, Sullivan PF, Kendler KS: Medical and psychiatric morbidity in obese women with and without binge eating. Int J Eat Disord 2002;32:72–78.

41   Devlin MJ, Goldfein JA, Dobrow I: What is this thing called BED? Current status of binge eating disorder nosology. Int J Eat Disord 2003;34:S2–S18.

42   Walsh BT, Boudreau G: Laboratory studies of binge eating disorder. Int J Eat Disord 2003;34: S30–S38.

43   Cooper Z, Fairburn CG: Refining the definition of binge eating disorder and nonpurging bulimia nervosa. Int J Eat Disord 2003;34:S89–S95.

44   Hay P, Fairburn CG: The validity of the DSM-IV scheme for classifying bulimic eating disorders. Int Eat Disord 1998;23:7–15.

45   Jacobi C, Paul T, de Zwaan M, Nutzinger DO, Dahme B: Specificity of self-concept disturbances in eating disorders. Int J Eat Disord 2004;35:204–210.

46   Wilfley DE, Welch RR, Stein RI, Spurrell EB, Cohen LR, Saelens BE, Dounchis JZ, Frank MA, Wiseman CV, Matt GE: A randomized comparison of group cognitive-behavioral therapy and group interpersonal psychotherapy for the treatment of overweight individuals with binge-eating disorder. Arch Gen Psychiatry 2002;59:713–721.

47   Wilson CT, Fairburn CG: Eating Disorders; in Nathan PE, Gorman M (eds): A Guide to Treatments that Work. New York, Oxford University Press, 2002, pp 559–592.

48   Fairburn CG, Jones R, Peveler RC, Carr S, Solomon R, O'Connor M, Burton J, Hope RC: Three psychological treatments for bulimia nervosa. A comparative trial. Arch Gen Psychiatry 1991;48: 463–469.

49   Agras S, Walsh BT, Fairburn CG, Wilson GT, Kraemer HC: A multicenter comparison of cognitive-behavioral therapy and interpersonal psychotherapy for bulimia nervosa. Arch Gen Psychiatry 2000;57:459–466.

50   Fairburn CG, Cooper Z, Doll HA, Norman P, O'Connor M: The natural course of bulimia nervosa and binge eating disorder in young women. Arch Gen Psychiatry 2000;57:659–665.

51   Smith DE, Marcus MD, Lewis CE, Fitzgibbon M, Schreiner P: Prevalence of binge eating disorder, obesity, and depression in a biracial cohort of young adults. Ann Behav Med 1998;20: 227–232.

52   Striegel-Moore RH, Wilfley DE, Pike KM, Dohm FA, Fairburn CG: Recurrent binge eating in Black American women. Arch Fam Med 2000;9:83–87.

53   Grilo CM: Binge eating disorder; in Fairburn CG, Brownell K (eds): Eating Disorders and Obesity: A Comprehensive Handbook, ed 2. New York, Guilford Press, 2000, pp 178–182.

54   Yanovski SZ, Nelson JE, Dubbert BK, Spitzer RL: Association of binge eating disorder and psychiatric comorbidity in obese subjects. Am J Psychiatry 1993;150:1472–1479.

Brunna Tuschen-Caffier, PhD
Department of Psychology, University of Bielefeld
Postfach 10 01 31, DE–33619 Bielefeld (Germany)
Tel. +49 0 521 1064493, Fax +49 0 521 106 89012
E-Mail brunna.tuschen@uni-bielefeld.de

Munsch S, Beglinger C (eds): Obesity and Binge Eating Disorder.
Bibl Psychiatr. Basel, Karger, 2005, No 171, pp 149–164

....

Course, Etiology, and Maintenance of Binge Eating Disorder

Anja Hilbert

Department of Psychiatry, School of Medicine,
Washington University, St. Louis, Mo., USA

Binge eating disorder (BED) is an eating disorder associated with clinically significant eating disorder and general psychopathology as well as impairments in psychosocial functioning and overall quality of life and is usually co-occurring with, yet distinct from, obesity [1–4]. Its inclusion in the DSM-IV as a provisional diagnosis in need of further study [5] has stimulated research on the clinical presentation, pathogenesis, and maintenance of this disorder. This chapter reviews clinically relevant research on the onset and course, etiology, and maintenance of BED.

Onset and Course

Studies subtyping the onset of BED identified two different patterns of development that may be associated with a distinctive clinical profile: Unlike individuals with bulimia nervosa, who usually start dieting before the onset of binge eating [6, 7], a relatively large number of individuals with BED report onset of binge eating prior to their first attempt at dieting (binge-first: 35–55%) [8–11]. In these patients, binge eating emerges at 11–13 years, which is significantly earlier than in those whose dieting precedes the first occurrence of binge eating (diet-first: 39–65%; onset of binge eating: 25–26 years). The binge-first group has been found to be more frequently associated with an earlier onset of overweight and BED diagnosis, a history of more psychiatric problems, higher rates of Axis II personality disorders, and higher frequency of exposure to weight-related critical comments. Early age of binge eating onset was further identified as a negative prognostic indicator for treatment success through psychological therapy [12, 13]; similarly, patients of the binge-first subtype were less than half as likely as patients of the diet-first group to be abstinent from binge eating 12 months after termination of psychological treatment [Wilfley et al., unpubl. data]. Of note, patterns of onset of binge eating and dieting were retrospectively assessed with most of the studies investigating Caucasian women seeking treatment, which may limit the reliability and generalizability of findings. Additional studies are needed for confirmation of binge-first vs. diet-first subtypes, using prospective designs and community samples of BED.

The natural course of BED is controversial mainly because of the ambiguity regarding stability and rates of spontaneous remission of the disorder. Some prospective studies show persistence of BED symptomatology, while others suggest a tendency to remit over time. One small community-based course study found that half of the participants met full BED criteria at the end of a 6-month follow-up (52%) while the other half was in partial remission; none of the participants was free of eating disorder symptoms at a 6-month follow-up [14]. A larger community-based study investigating the 5-year course of BED found only 18% affected from some form of clinical eating disorder after 5 years [15]. Of note, the prevalence of obesity in those presenting with BED at baseline had almost doubled after 5 years, indicating that BED may be a risk factor for future weight gain. One-year follow-up results from the largest community-based study of eating disorders to date showed a much higher degree of stability, with the majority of individuals with BED having either full or partial BED at 1-year follow-up (64%), and only 7% presenting without any eating disorder diagnosis [16]. A clinical follow-up study of BED found that 6 years following inpatient treatment, 6% were still affected by BED, 7% were diagnosed as having an eating disorder not otherwise specified (EDNOS), 7% had developed bulimia nervosa, and the remainder did not have an eating disorder as defined in the DSM-IV [17]. The heterogeneity of the results may be due to differences in age and duration of illness in the populations assessed; for example, the studies by Fairburn et al. [15] and Fichter et al. [17] investigated individuals at young age and short duration of illness, which may account for a higher tendency of remission than found by other studies. In clinical settings, however, patients with BED frequently report a long history of the disorder, and it is thus plausible that BED has a fluctuating course, marked by intermittent remission and resurgence of symptoms. Future research is needed in order to clarify the natural course of BED.

Etiology

Increasing evidence suggests that BED may be understood as a multifactorial condition resulting from genetic, psychological, and social factors. First, the empirical status of risk factor research in BED will be described, followed by an outline of theoretical models for explanation of interactions between risk factors in the development of BED.

A small number of studies have investigated the genetic transmission of binge eating and BED, respectively. Family studies have provided mixed evidence of a familial aggregation of BED in female samples, presumably due to small sample sizes [18, 19]. A population-based study on female twins from the Virginia Twin Registry revealed a moderate heritability for binge eating (49%) and a substantial heritability for obesity (86%). Genetic overlap between risk factors for both traits was modest [20]. Analyses from a Norwegian population-based twin registry found a similar magnitude of genetic and environmental effects on binge eating for males and females, suggesting equal heritability (51%), and mainly shared genetic risk factors in both sexes [21]. Molecular-genetic findings indicating that binge eating may be caused by mutations in the melanocortin-4 receptor gene [22] were not replicated yet [23]. Overall, results are suggestive of a genetic basis of binge eating. However, since the number of studies is small and DSM-IV research criteria of BED were frequently not applied, the heritability of BED remains largely unknown.

Two comprehensive studies on psychosocial risk factors of BED have been performed [24; (Striegel-Moore et al., unpubl. data]. In a community-based case-control study, Fairburn and colleagues conducted a retrospective risk factor interview with women with BED. Compared to a control group without eating or other psychiatric disorders, women with BED revealed greater exposure to certain adverse childhood experiences (e.g., sexual or physical abuse, bullying); family problems (e.g., parental psychiatric disorder, parental criticism, lack of affection, underinvolvement or overprotection); and negative comments about shape, weight, and eating. Childhood psychosocial vulnerability (e.g., negative self-evaluation, shyness) also increased the risk for later development of BED. Compared to a non-eating-disordered psychiatric control group, the BED group reported significantly higher rates of childhood obesity and negative comments about shape, weight, and eating, suggesting that these risk factors may be specific for BED in comparison with those for other psychiatric disorders. Participants with BED reported similar exposure to specific risk factors as participants with bulimia nervosa, but an overall lower personal vulnerability, particularly of childhood and parental obesity. Results from the New England Women's Health Project (NEWHP) using a similar design and methodology mainly confirmed findings on psychosocial risk factors of BED [Striegel-Moore et al., in press]. For example, women with BED and psychiatric control women reported higher rates of exposure to negative affect, parental mood and substance disorders, perfectionism, separation from parents, and maternal problems than non-psychiatric control women. In addition, findings from the NEWHP emphasize the importance of familial factors as specific risk factors in the pathogenesis of BED by indicating greater exposure to familial eating problems, family discord, high parental demands, and childhood obesity in BED than in psychiatric disorders. Race did not appear to moderate risk for BED. Overall, these results suggest that a variety of life events, familial problems, and personal vulnerability factors increases the risk of developing BED. However, given that psychosocial risk factor research in BED is based on retrospective assessment, precedence of risk factors to the onset of disordered eating cannot clearly be established, and thus, risk factor status remains to be confirmed in prospective designs [25, 26].

Prospective risk factor studies in the field of eating disorders have mostly investigated the development of bulimic symptomatology (i.e. binge eating and purging), but not of BED [27]. Among the few risk factor studies prospectively examining binge eating separately from inappropriate compensatory behaviors, a two-year prospective study by Stice and colleagues identified several independent risk factors for the development of self-reported binge eating in female adolescents, including elevated dieting, pressure to be thin, modeling of eating disturbances, appearance overevaluation, body dissatisfaction, depressive symptoms, emotional eating, body mass, and low self-esteem and social support [28]. Binge eating was not only predicted by elevated body mass, but also predicted onset of obesity. An analysis of interactions between risk factors showed an increased risk for girls who overevaluated appearance, had an elevated body mass index (BMI; in kg/m^2), and dieted (42%). Another four-year prospective study identified restrained eating and negative affect as predictors for binge eating in female adolescents with the highest risk at age 16 [29]. Since these prospective studies did not apply the research criteria of BED, thereby not excluding individuals with inappropriate compensatory behaviors, it is unclear to what extent the findings are generalizable to BED.

In summary, a number of psychological, social, and biological risk factors may contribute to the development of binge eating and BED. It is, however, not known through which psychobiological mechanisms these putative risk factors and antecedents interact in the pathogenesis of BED, e.g., how obesity, dieting, and binge eating mutually influence each other. The previously described results of binge-first vs. dieting-first subtypes of eating pathology onset (see Onset and Course) permit speculation of different etiological pathways leading to BED. While restraint (i.e. dietary restriction and/or dietary restraint)[1] may be a risk

---

[1]The concept of restraint has been operationalized in various ways, frequently distinguishing the components of dietary restriction vs. dietary restraint [30]. Here, dietary restriction indicates the actual restriction of food intake for shape and weight reasons (i.e. actual dieting, restrictive eating patterns), whereas dietary restraint describes the intent to diet and attempts to restrict food intake for shape and weight reasons (e.g., attempts to follow dietary rules or avoid 'fattening' foods).

---

factor for binge eating in the diet-first subgroup, which would conform to empirical findings on bulimia nervosa [26], in the binge-first group, binge eating seems to develop more against a background of psychiatric symptomatology [9]. Thus, the restraint model developed for bulimia nervosa positing that restraint increases the likelihood of binge eating [31] may apply only to a subgroup of individuals with BED. The overall decreased impact of restraint on the development of binge eating in BED is consistent with findings from controlled trials on behavioral weight loss, which show that caloric restriction does not increase binge eating in the short term, and is as effective as cognitive-behavioral psychotherapy to reduce binge eating [32–34] [see chapter by Biedert, this vol., pp 165–179]; long-term effects of dietary restriction, however, are not yet established [35].

Several theoretical models have been elaborated to explain interactions between risk factors in the development of binge eating. A comprehensive framework that combines theoretical accounts of sociocultural [36], dietary [31], and affect regulation factors [37] is the dual-pathway model proposed by Stice and Agras [38]. Although designed and evaluated as an etiological model of bulimic pathology including binge eating and purging, the dual-pathway model includes many determinants that are putative risk factors for the development of BED (e.g., restraint, negative self-evaluation, and critical comments about shape and weight). The dual-pathway model postulates that body dissatisfaction is fostered by sociocultural pressure to be thin and an internalized thin ideal. Through two pathways, either of which being sufficient, body dissatisfaction may contribute to the development of bulimic pathology: In the restraint pathway, body dissatisfaction accounts for restraint; restraint in turn increases the likelihood of binge eating as a response to caloric restriction and/or the breaking of strict dietary rules ('abstinence violation effect'). In the affect regulation pathway, body dissatisfaction provokes negative affect because appearance becomes a central aspect of negative self-evaluation. Negative affect can also be promoted by dieting because of the impact of caloric deprivation on negative mood and/or because of failure that is often associated with unsuccessful dieting attempts. Binge eating is used for coping with negative affect, e.g., by providing comfort and/or distraction from negative affect; likewise, purging may be used for affect regulation purposes. The dual-pathway model was cross-sectionally [39, 40] and prospectively validated in adolescent girls and young women [41, 42], but since DSM-IV research criteria of BED were not applied, it still needs to be ascertained whether the model is predictive of the development of BED, especially because of the unclear role of restraint in the etiology of this disorder [31]. Another etiological model specifically developed for the explanation of the pathogenesis of BED, the integrated model of risk for BED [43], focuses on the developmental stages earlier than adolescence emphasized by the dual-pathway model. The integrated model of risk for BED combines accounts from restraint theory and interpersonal theory. In the inter-personal vulnerability component (for the restraint component, see above), family problems (e.g., parental psychopathology, criticism, neglect, lack of affection) and abusive experiences are assumed to cause disturbances in early child-caretaker relationships that lead to the development of a vulnerable self (e.g., low self-esteem) exhibiting interpersonal (e.g., social concerns, loneli-ness) and affect regulation difficulties (e.g., difficulties in coping with negative emotions in response to life stress). Binge eating is understood as an attempt to manage these adverse affective experiences. Determinants of the interpersonal vulnerability model are consistent with risk factor research (see above), find-ings on impaired interpersonal functioning in BED [44, 45], and effectiveness of interpersonal psychotherapy, a therapeutic approach focusing on interper-sonal problems in significant relationships [46, 47] [see chapter by Biedert, this vol., pp 165–179]. The etiological cascade of the interpersonal vulnerability model, however, awaits empirical validation.

Maintenance

The following section reviews findings on biological, psychological, behavioral, and environmental factors and theoretical models of the mainte-nance of binge eating in BED.

Biological Factors

There is little evidence for biological correlates of binge eating in BED [for biological factors related to obesity, see chapter by Vögele, this vol., pp 62–73]. As compared to weight-matched controls, obese individuals with BED or obese binge eaters, respectively, did not show abnormalities in:

- metabolism, e.g., serum insulin, triglyceride, cholesterol, and thyroid hormones [48, 49];
- resting energy expenditure [50];
- cephalic phase response consisting of the first physical responses to the sight, smell, taste, or thought of food (e.g., serum insulin, glucose toler-ance, and salivation in response to food exposure) [51];
- hypothalamic-pituitary-adrenal function (e.g., dexamethasone suppression or cortisol and adrenocorticotropin response to corticotropin-releasing hormone) [52];
- serotonergic function involved in the modulation of feeding behavior, mood, and impulse control; no evidence was found for an altered central nervous system serotonin (5-HT) neurotransmitter activity in BED (e.g., prolactin response to D-fenfluramine) [53];

- leptin, a protein controlling hypothalamic pathways of energy metabolism; serum leptin levels were not altered in BED and unrelated to food intake, hunger, and the desire to eat in response to food stimuli [51, 54, 55];
- neuroactive steroid hormones assumed to modulate eating behavior (e.g., plasma levels of $3\alpha,5\alpha$-tetrahydroprogesterone, and dehydroepiandrosterone) [56].

The fact that BED, as opposed to anorexia nervosa and bulimia nervosa, is not associated with perturbations on the aforementioned biological parameters suggests that such disturbances are more likely associated with starvation, underweight status, purging behavior, and/or excessive exercising than with binge eating [52, 57]. Yet, a few recent studies using fine-grained functional brain imaging techniques, such as single-photon emission tomography, found reduced serotonin transporter binding in obese binge eaters compared to non-binge eaters, which may be related to increased hunger and food intake [58]. Further, when exposed to food cues, obese binge eaters showed a greater increase of the regional cerebral blood flow in the left than in the right hemisphere, especially in the frontal and pre-frontal regions, than obese non-binge eaters [59]. Significant associations between cerebral blood flow in the respective regions and increases of hunger during food exposure suggest that the left hemispheric frontal and pre-frontal regions may be involved in the maintenance of binge eating. Other studies have suggested a decreased satiety response in BED. Geliebter and Hashim [60] found that binge eating, not obesity, was associated with a higher gastric capacity, suggesting that binge eaters may need to consume larger quantities of food in order to feel satiation through gastric stretch or mechanoreceptors than weight-matched non-binge eaters. Thus, an increased stomach capacity, slower gastric emptying, and, relatedly, decreased release of cholecystokinin (a putative satiety hormone released in the duodenum) may perpetuate large food intake through decreased satiety responses. Further, Raymond et al. [61] found higher pain detection thresholds in obese women with BED than without BED. These higher thresholds were assumed to be related to vagal hypertonia, possibly maintaining binge eating through a reduced satiety response.

Restraint

The DSM-IV research criteria define BED primarily by recurrent episodes of binge eating in the absence of regular use of inappropriate compensatory behavior such as fasting. In accordance with these criteria, individuals with BED exhibit less dietary restriction than non-BED individuals. Obese individuals with BED consumed significantly more calories than obese individuals without BED when instructions for 'normal' and binge eating were given under structured laboratory conditions [62], and consumed significantly more liquid meal during a 24-hour feeding paradigm [63]. In the natural environment, obese binge eaters self-monitored increased caloric intake on binge days, but moderate dietary restriction on non-binge days [64]. Accordingly, individuals with BED were found to maintain greater dietary restraint, i.e. more attempts at restricting food intake, on non-binge than on binge days [65]. Overall, individuals with BED report moderate levels of dietary restraint, which are higher than in the normal weight population, lower than in bulimia nervosa and anorexia nervosa, but similar to weight-matched non-BED obese [66–69]. Dietary restraint was found to be unrelated to binge eating frequency in obese outpatients with BED, but positively associated with eating disorder psychopathology (i.e. concerns on shape, weight, and eating), suggesting that dietary restraint does not impact binge eating directly, but indirectly via eating disorder psychopathology [70]. Based on these results, it cannot be ruled out that binge eating may be maintained by moderate dietary restriction and restraint. Yet binge eating clearly appears associated with a general tendency towards eating disinhibition, e.g., eating in response to emotional or external cues [48, 66, 71], overeating habits, and chaotic eating patterns. For example, obese individuals reported binge eating problems frequently in association with 'grazing,' a pattern of recurrent subjective episodes of binge eating (as defined as consumption of an ordinary amount of food, accompanied by a sense of loss of control over eating) [72].

Negative Mood

Negative mood is presumably the most well-established antecedent of binge eating in BED, with support from studies using retrospective [71, 73–76] and concurrent self-report [77–79] as well as experimental designs [80, 81]. To highlight some of the findings, a study utilizing handheld computers for the assessment of daily eating behavior in the naturalistic setting ('ecological momentary assessment' technology) [82], found obese individuals with BED to experience more negative mood prior to binge eating than obese individuals with subclinical binge eating, and mood was lower prior to binge eating than prior to regular episodes of eating or independent from eating [78]. Further antecedents of binge eating in BED were low alertness, feelings of low control over eating, and craving sweets. An experimental study investigated the effects of negative mood induction and caloric deprivation on binge eating in obese women with BED [81]. The combination of negative mood and caloric deprivation increased the occurrence of objective episodes of binge eating (as defined by consumption of an unambiguously large amount of food, accompanied by loss of control over eating; see DSM-IV). Negative mood, but not caloric deprivation, increased subjectively perceived binge eating (defined above). These results suggest that both negative mood and dietary restriction account for binge eating pathology in BED. Here, dietary restriction appears to potentiate the triggering effect of negative mood on loss of control over eating.

Negative mood may be particularly important as a maintaining factor in a subgroup of individuals with BED. Subtyping of BED women along dietary restraint and negative affect dimensions showed a low negative affect subtype (LNA; 64–70% of cases) and a high negative affect subtype (HNA; 30–36% of cases), both associated with moderate levels of dietary restraint and relatively stable over time [83–85]. The HNA subtype is characterized by significantly greater eating disorder and general psychopathology (e.g., more eating, weight, and shape concerns; more comorbid and/or lifetime depressive disorders; higher levels of associated psychiatric disturbance and social maladjustment). Both the HNA and the LNA subtypes may be maintained by moderate levels of restraint; individuals with HNA may additionally make greater use of binge eating as a measure of affect regulation [37]. Consistently, the fact that patients of the HNA subtype reveal poorer outcome after cognitive-behavioral self-help treatment than patients of the LNA subtype [85] suggests that such additional maintaining mechanisms may be in place, making the HNA subtype more resistant to change than the LNA subtype. Of note, in addition to negative mood states, positive mood states were found to be associated with binge eating episodes. For example, compared to women with bulimia nervosa, overweight women with BED reported greater enjoyment while consuming binge food and less negative consequences following binge eating episodes (e.g., physical discomfort) [75], suggesting that hedonics may play a role as maintaining factors of binge eating in BED.

Body Image Disturbance
Body image disturbance presents against a sociocultural background that idealizes thinness and physical fitness and simultaneously stigmatizes overweight and obesity [86]. Individuals with BED exhibit a body image disturbance that is as severe as in bulimia nervosa; specifically, individuals with BED are strongly concerned with body shape and weight, over-evaluate the importance of shape and weight, and reveal more negative body-related thinking, body dissatisfaction, feelings of fatness, and discomfort with and avoidance of seeing one's body as compared to weight-matched individuals without eating disorders [68, 71, 87–92]. Body image disturbance appears to result from eating disorder psychopathology rather than from obese body weight, since patients with BED present similarly on shape and weight concerns, irrespective of their degree of overweight [71]. Using structural equation modeling, shape and weight concerns were identified as maintaining factors of binge eating in individuals with BED [93] and there is evidence that over-evaluation

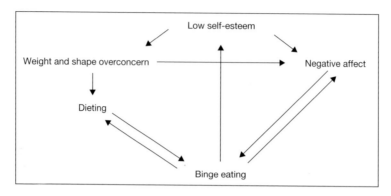

Fig. 1. Cognitive-behavioral model of the maintenance of binge eating disorder (with permission from [1]).

of shape and weight is associated with less spontaneous recovery in BED over a six-month follow-up period [14].

Environmental and Other Psychosocial Factors

As evidenced by experimental test meal studies, obese individuals with BED consume more food and energy when greater number and quantities of foods are available [94, 95]. This tendency to eat in response to food cues may be mediated by a subjective desire to eat: when exposed to food cues, obese binge eaters experienced greater subjective desire to eat than obese non-binge eaters [51, 96], suggesting that an increased subjective reactivity to food cues likely contributes to the maintenance of binge eating.

There is further evidence that experience of daily stress, but not the number of stressors, is a precursor of binge eating [79, 97].

Cognitive-Behavioral Model of BED

Several theoretical models have been developed to explain the maintenance of binge eating, the most clinically relevant of which may be the cognitive-behavioral model. Originally developed for bulimia nervosa [98], Castonguay et al. [1] adapted it to BED by considering the impact of being overweight, a lesser role of restraint, and negative mood as a trigger of binge eating (fig. 1). In this cognitive-behavioral model of BED, low self-esteem is seen as giving rise to weight and shape overconcern and negative affect. Weight and shape overconcern increases motivation to diet. Binge eating is partially consequence of physiological and cognitive mechanisms related to dieting. Also, binge eating occurs as an avoidance coping response to negative affect which is increased by low self-esteem. Detrimental effects of binge eating on mood and self-esteem and compensatory dieting efforts perpetuate this vicious cycle. An empirical test of the cognitive-behavioral model confirmed most of the postulated associations within the model using structural equation modeling [93]. As opposed to the model, weight and shape overconcern directly predicted binge eating, while both restraint and negative affect were influenced by shape and weight overconcern, but were not significantly associated with binge eating. These results underline the central role of body image disturbance as a maintaining factor of binge eating in BED. Additionally, this study found low self-esteem to be predicted by high levels of perfectionism (e.g., perceived pressure to conform to unrealistically high expectations from others). Consistently, a recent extension of the cognitive-behavioral model of bulimia nervosa by Fairburn and colleagues [99], the transdiagnostic theory, conceptualizes clinical perfectionism as an additional maintaining factor of eating disorder psychopathology. The transdiagnostic theory assumes that the psychopathology of BED, bulimia nervosa, anorexia nervosa, and other EDNOS is maintained by similar psychopathological processes and that additional mechanisms complicate the maintenance of the psychopathology of certain eating disordered patients. Other additional mechanisms that may occur in BED are core low self-esteem, a fundamental and global negative view of oneself; mood intolerance, i.e. inability to effectively regulate both negative and positive mood states, and interpersonal difficulties that trigger binge eating episodes. Future research will need to comprehensively test the postulated maintaining mechanisms of binge eating in BED.

Conclusion

Since BED was defined as a psychiatric disorder in need of further study, research has substantially increased knowledge on course, etiology, and maintenance of this disorder. BED presents as a complex condition that is presumably determined and maintained by multiple biological, psychological, and social factors, associated with and likely increasing the risk of obesity. Table 1 summarizes current knowledge about course, etiology, and maintenance of the disorder.

Challenges for future research include further understanding hereditary and psychosocial risk factors of BED and the mechanisms of interaction between these factors; psychobiological correlates of binge eating and feeding behavior; the natural course of BED, especially regarding stability and tendency of spontaneous remission; and the relationship between binge eating and obesity in the development of BED. Since most of the studies to date have been conducted on Caucasian females, future investigations will need to explicitly

Table 1. Current knowledge on onset, course, etiology, and maintenance of BED

Onset	35–55% of patients with BED start binge eating prior to their first attempt at dieting (onset of binge eating: 11–13 years), while 39–65% report dieting prior to first occurrence of binge eating (onset of binge eating: 25–26 years)
Course	Controversial regarding stability and rates of spontaneous remission
Etiology	Barely studied genetic basis of BED; putative psychosocial risk factors include childhood psychosocial vulnerability, adverse childhood experiences, family problems, negative comments about shape, weight, and eating; unclear nature of relationship between binge eating and obesity
Maintenance	Little evidence on biological maintaining factors of binge eating in BED; maintaining factors of binge eating include weight and shape concerns, negative affect, food stimuli, and stressful experiences

include male and racial or ethnic minority samples. Enhancing knowledge on course, etiology, and maintenance of BED is essential not only to clarify the nosological status of this disorder [100], but also to refine empirically informed approaches to treatment and prevention.

References

1 Castonguay LG, Eldredge KL, Agras WS: Binge eating disorder: Current state and future directions. Clin Psychol Rev 1995;15:865–890.
2 de Zwaan M: Binge eating disorder and obesity. Int J Obes 2001;25:S51–S55.
3 Dingemans AE, Bruna MJ, van Furth EF: Binge eating disorder: A review. Int J Obes 2002;26: 299–307.
4 Wilfley DE, Wilson GT, Agras, WS: The clinical significance of binge eating disorder. Int J Eat Disord 2003;34:S96–S106.
5 American Psychiatric Association: Diagnostic and Statistical Manual of Mental Disorders, ed 4, revised, 1994.
6 Mussell MP, Mitchell JE, Fenna CJ, Crosby RD, Miller JP, Hoberman HM: A comparison of onset of binge eating versus dieting in the development of bulimia nervosa. Int J Eat Disord 1997;21:353–360.
7 Haiman C, Devlin MJ: Binge eating before the onset of dieting: A distinct subgroup of bulimia nervosa? Int J Eat Disord 1999;25:151–157.
8 Mussell MP, Mitchell JE, Weller CL, Raymond NC, Crow SJ, Crosby RD: Onset of binge eating, dieting, obesity, and mood disorders among subjects seeking treatment for binge eating disorder. Int J Eat Disord 1995;17:395–401.
9 Spurrell EB, Wilfley DE, Tanofsky MB, Brownell KD: Age of onset for binge eating: Are there different pathways to binge eating? Int J Eat Disord 1997;21:55–65.
10 Abbott DW, de Zwaan M, Mussell MP, Raymond NC, Seim HC, Crow SJ, Crosby RD, Mitchell JE: Onset of binge eating and dieting in overweight women: Implications for etiology, associated features and treatment. J Psychosom Res 1998;44:367–374.
11 Grilo CM, Masheb RM: Onset of dieting vs. binge eating in outpatients with binge eating disorder. Int J Obes 2000;24:404–409.
12 Agras WS, Telch CF, Arnow B, Eldredge K, Detzer MJ, Henderson J, Marnell M: Does interpersonal therapy help patients with binge eating disorder who fail to respond to cognitive-behavioral therapy? J Consult Clin Psychol 1995;63:356–360.

13 Safer DL, Lively TJ, Telch CF, Agras WS: Predictors of relapse following successful dialectical behavior therapy for binge eating disorder. Int J Eat Disord 2002;32:155–163.

14 Cachelin FM, Striegel-Moore RH, Elder KA, Pike KM, Wilfley DE, Fairburn CG: Natural course of a community sample of women with binge eating disorder. Int J Eat Disord 1999;25:45–54.

15 Fairburn CG, Cooper Z, Doll HA, Norman P, O'Connor M: The natural course of bulimia nervosa and binge eating disorder in young women. Arch Gen Psychiatry 2000;57:659–665.

16 Crow SJ, Agras WS, Halmi K, Mitchell JE, Kraemer HC: Full syndromal versus subthreshold anorexia nervosa, bulimia nervosa, and binge eating disorder: A multicenter study. Int J Eat Disord 2002;32:309–318.

17 Fichter MM, Quadflieg N, Gnutzmann A: Binge eating disorder: Treatment outcome over a 6-year course. J Psychosom Res 1998;44:385–405.

18 Fowler SJ, Bulik CM: Family environment and psychiatric history in women with binge eating disorder and obese controls. Behav Change 1997;14:106–112.

19 Lee YH, Abbott DW, Seim H, Crosby RD, Monson N, Burgard M, Mitchell JE: Eating disorders and psychiatric disorders in the first-degree relatives of obese probands with binge eating disorder and obese non-binge eating disorder controls. Int J Eat Disord 1999;26:322–332.

20 Bulik CM, Sullivan PF, Kendler KS: Genetic and environmental contributions to obesity and binge eating. Int J Eat Disord 2003;33:293–298.

21 Reichborn-Kjennerud T, Bulik CM, Kendler KS, Roysamb E, Maes H, Tambs K, Harris JR: Gender differences in binge-eating: A population-based twin study. Acta Psychiatr Scand 2003;108:196–202.

22 Branson R, Potoczna N, Kral JG, Lentes KU, Hoehe MR, Horber FF: Binge eating as a major phenotype of melanocortin 4 receptor gene mutations. N Engl J Med 2003;348:1096–1103.

23 Hebebrand J, Geller F, Dempfle A, Heinzel-Gutenbrunner M, Raab M, Gerber G, Wermter AK, Horro FF, Blundell J, Schäfer H, Remschmidt H, Herpertz S, Hinney A: Binge eating episodes are not characteristic of carriers of melanocortin-4 receptor gene mutations. Mol Psychiatry 2004; Epub ahead of print:1–5.

24 Fairburn CG, Doll HA, Welch SL, Hay PJ, Davies BA, O'Connor ME: Risk factors for binge eating disorder: A community-based, case-control study. Arch Gen Psychiatry 1998;55:425–432.

25 Kraemer HC, Kazdin AE, Offord DR, Kessler RC, Jensen PS, Kupfer DJ: Coming to terms with the terms of risk. Arch Gen Psychiatry 1997;54:337–343.

26 Jacobi C, Hayward C, de Zwaan M, Kraemer HC, Agras WS: Coming to terms with risk factors for eating disorders: Application of risk terminology and suggestions for a general taxonomy. Psychol Bull 2004;130:19–65.

27 Stice E: Risk and maintenance factors for eating pathology: A meta-analytic review. Psychol Bull 2002;128:825–848.

28 Stice E, Presnell K, Spangler D: Risk factors for binge eating onset in adolescent girls: A 2-year prospective investigation. Health Psychol 2002;21:131–138.

29 Stice E, Killen JD, Hayward C, Taylor CB: Age of onset for binge eating and purging during late adolescence: A 4-year survival analysis. J Abnorm Psychol 1998;107:671–675.

30 Howard CE, Porzelius LK: The role of dieting in binge eating disorder: Etiology and treatment implications. Clin Psychol Rev 1999;19:25–44.

31 Polivy J, Herman CP: Dieting and binging: A causal analysis. Am Psychol 1985;40:193–201.

32 Marcus MD, Wing RR, Fairburn CG: Cognitive behavioral treatment of binge eating vs. behavioral weight control on the treatment of binge eating disorder. Ann Behav Med 1995;17:S090.

33 Nauta H, Hospers H, Kok G, Jansen A: A comparison between a cognitive and a behavioral treatment for obese binge eaters and obese non-binge eaters. Behav Ther 2000;31:441–461.

34 Agras WS, Telch CF, Arnow B, Eldredge K, Wilfley DE, Raeburn SD, Henderson J, Marnell M: Weight loss, cognitive behavioral, and desipramine treatments in binge eating disorder: An additive design. Behav Ther 1994;25:225–238.

35 Nauta H, Hospers H, Jansen A: One-year follow-up effects of two obesity treatments on psychological well-being and weight. Br J Health Psychol 2001;6:271–284.

36 Striegel-Moore RH, Silberstein LR, Rodin J: Toward an understanding of risk factors for bulimia. Am Psychol 1986;41:246–263.

37 Heatherton TF, Baumeister RF: Binge eating as escape from self awareness. Psychol Bull 1991;110:86–108.

38   Stice E, Agras WS: Predicting onset and cessation bulimic behaviors during adolescence: A longitudinal grouping analysis. Behav Ther 1998;29:257–276.

39   Stice E, Nemeroff C, Shaw HE: Test of the dual pathway model of bulimia nervosa: Evidence for dietary restraint and affect regulation mechanisms. J Soc Clin Psychol 1996;15:340–363.

40   Ricciardelli LA, McCabe MP: Dietary restraint and negative affect as mediators of body dissatisfaction and bulimic behavior in adolescent girls and boys. Behav Res Ther 2001;39:1317–1328.

41   Stice E, Shaw H, Nemeroff C: Dual pathway model of bulimia nervosa: Longitudinal support for dietary restraint and affect-regulation mechanisms. J Soc Clin Psychol 1998;17:129–149.

42   Stice E: A prospective test of the dual-pathway model of bulimic pathology: Mediating effects of dieting and negative affect. J Abnorm Psychol 2001;110:124–135.

43   Wilfley DE, Pike KM, Striegel-Moore RH: Toward an integrated model of risk for binge eating disorder. J Gend Cult Health 1997;2:1–32.

44   Fassino S, Leombruni P, Pierò A, Abbate-Daga G, Rovera GG: Mood, eating attitudes, and anger in obese women with and without binge eating disorder. J Psychosom Res 2003;54:559–566.

45   Friedman MA, Wilfley DE, Welch RR, Kunce JT: Self-directed hostility and family functioning in normal-weight bulimics and overweight binge eaters. Addict Behav 1997;22:367–375.

46   Wilfley DE, Agras WS, Telch CF, Rossiter EM, Schneider JA, Cole AG, Sifford LA, Raeburn SD: Group cognitive-behavioral therapy and group interpersonal psychotherapy for the nonpurging bulimic individual: A controlled comparison. J Consul Clin Psychol 1993;61:296–305.

47   Wilfley DE, Welch RR, Stein RI, Spurrell EB, Cohen LR, Saelens BE, Dounchis JZ, Frank MA, Wiseman CV, Matt GE: A randomized comparison of group cognitive-behavioral therapy and group interpersonal psychotherapy for the treatment of overweight individuals with binge-eating disorder. Arch Gen Psychiatry 2002;59:713–721.

48   Wadden TA, Foster GD, Letizia KA, Wilk JE: Metabolic, anthropometric, and psychological characteristics of obese binge eaters. Int J Eat Disord 1993;14:17–25.

49   Adami GF, Gandolfo P, Campostano A, Cocchi F, Bauer B, Scopinaro N: Obese binge eaters: Metabolic characteristics, energy expenditure and dieting. Psychol Med 1995;25:195–198.

50   de Zwaan M, Aslam Z, Mitchell JE: Research on energy expenditure in individuals with eating disorders: A review. Int J Eat Disord 2002;32:127–134.

51   Karhunen LJ, Lappalainen RI, Tammela L, Turpeinen AK, Uusitupa MI: Subjective and physiological cephalic phase responses to food in obese binge-eating women. Int J Eat Disord 1997;21:321–328.

52   Yanovski SZ: Biological correlates of binge eating. Addict Behav 1995;20:705–712.

53   Monteleone P, Brambilla F, Bortolotti F, Maj M: Serotonergic dysfunction across the eating disorders: Relationship to eating behaviour, purging behaviour, nutritional status and general psychopathology. Psychol Med 2000;30:1099–1110.

54   Adami G, Campostano A, Cella F, Ferrandes G: Serum leptin level and restrained eating: Study with the Eating Disorder Examination. Physiol Behav 2002;75:189–192.

55   Monteleone P, Fabrazzo M, Tortorella A, Fuschino A, Maj M: Opposite modifications in circulating leptin and soluble leptin receptor across the eating disorder spectrum. Mol Psychiatry 2002;7:641–646.

56   Monteleone P, Luisi M, De Filippis G, Colurcio B, Monteleone P, Genazzani AR, Maj M: Circulating levels of neuroactive steroids in patients with binge eating disorder: A comparison with nonobese healthy controls and non-binge eating obese subjects. Int J Eat Disord 2003;34:432–440.

57   Halmi KA: Physiology of anorexia nervosa and bulimia nervosa; in Fairburn CG, Brownell KD (eds): Eating Disorders and Obesity. New York, Guilford Press, 2002, pp 293–297.

58   Kuikka JT, Tammela L, Karhunen L, Rissanen A, Bergström KA, Naukkarinen H, Vanninen E, Karhu J, Lappalainen R, Repo-Tiihonen E, Tiihonen J, Uusitupa MI: Reduced serotonin transporter binding in binge eating women. Psychopharmacology 2001;155:310–314.

59   Karhunen LJ, Vanninen EJ, Kuikka JT, Lappalainen RI, Tiihonen J, Uusitupa MIJ: Regional cerebral blood flow during exposure to food in obese binge eating women. Psychiatry Res 2000;99:29–42.

60   Geliebter A, Hashim SA: Gastric capacity in normal, obese, and bulimic women. Physiol Behav 2001;74:743–746.

61   Raymond NC, de Zwaan M, Faris PL, Nugent SM, Ackard DM, Crosby RD, Mitchell JE: Pain thresholds in obese binge-eating disorder subjects. Biol Psychiatry 1995;37:202–204.

62 Walsh BT, Boudreau G: Laboratory studies of binge eating disorder. Int J Eat Disord 2003;34:S30–S38.

63 Hsu LK, Mulliken B, McDonagh B, Krupa Das S, Rand W, Fairburn CG, Rolls B, McCrory MA, Saltzman E, Shikora S, Dwyer J, Roberts S: Binge eating disorder in extreme obesity. Int J Obes Relat Metab Disord 2002;26:1398–1403.

64 Rossiter EM, Agras WS, Telch CF, Bruce B: The eating patterns of non purging bulimic subjects. Int J Eat Disord 1992;11:111–120.

65 Eldredge KL, Agras WS: Instability of restraint among clinical binge eaters: A methodological note. Int J Eat Disord 1994;15:285–287.

66 Brody ML, Walsh BT, Devlin MJ: Binge eating disorder: Reliability and validity of a new diagnostic category. J Consult Clin Psychol 1994;62:381–386.

67 Masheb RM, Grilo CM: Binge eating disorder: A need for additional diagnostic criteria. Compr Psychiatry 2000;41:159–162.

68 Wilfley DE, Schwartz MB, Spurrell EB, Fairburn CG: Using the Eating Disorder Examination to identify the specific psychopathology of binge eating disorder. Int J Eat Disord 2000;27:259–269.

69 de Zwaan M, Mitchell JE, Howell LM, Monson N, Swan-Kremeier L, Crosby RD, Seim HC: Characteristics of morbidly obese patients before gastric bypass surgery. Compr Psychiatry 2003;44:428–434.

70 Masheb RM, Grilo CM: On the relation of attempting to lose weight, restraint, and binge eating in outpatients with binge eating disorder. Obes Res 2000;8:638–645.

71 Eldredge KL, Agras WS: Weight and shape overconcern and emotional eating in binge eating disorder. Int J Eat Disord 1996;19:73–82.

72 Saunders R: Binge eating in gastric bypass patients before surgery. Obes Surg 1999;9:72–76.

73 Arnow B, Kenardy J, Agras WS: Binge eating among the obese: A descriptive study. J Behav Med 1992;15:155–170.

74 Tanofsky MB, Wilfley DE, Spurrell EB, Welch R, Brownell KD: Comparison of men and women with binge eating disorder. Int J Eat Disord 1997;21:49–54.

75 Mitchell JE, Mussell MP, Peterson CB, Crow S, Wonderlich SA, Crosby RD, Davis T, Weller C: Hedonics of binge eating in women with bulimia nervosa and binge eating disorder. Int J Eat Disord 1999;26:165–170.

76 Pinaquy S, Chabrol H, Simon C, Louvet JP, Barbe P: Emotional eating, alexithymia, and binge-eating disorder in obese women. Obes Res 2003;11:195–201.

77 Johnson WG, Schlundt DG, Barclay DR, Carr-Nangle RE, Engler LB: A naturalistic functional analysis of binge eating. Behav Ther 1995;26:101–118.

78 Greeno CG, Wing RR, Shiffman S: Binge antecedents in obese women with and without binge eating disorder. J Consult Clin Psychol 2000;68:95–102.

79 le Grange D, Gorin A, Catley D, Stone AA: Does momentary assessment detect binge eating in overweight women that is denied at interview? Eur Eat Disord Rev 2001;9:309–324.

80 Telch CF, Agras WS: Do emotional states influence binge eating in the obese? Int J Eat Disord 1996;20:271–279.

81 Agras WS, Telch CF: The effects of caloric deprivation and negative affect on binge eating in obese binge-eating disordered women. Behav Ther 1998;29:491–503.

82 Stone AA, Shiffman S: Ecological momentary assessment (EMA) in behavorial medicine. Ann Behav Med 1994;16:199–202.

83 Stice E, Agras WS, Telch CF, Halmi KA, Mitchell JE, Wilson T: Subtyping binge eating-disordered women along dieting and negative affect dimensions. Int J Eat Disord 2001;30:11–27.

84 Grilo CM, Masheb RM, Wilson GT: Subtyping binge eating disorder. J Consult Clin Psychol 2001;69:1066–1072.

85 Loeb KL, Wilson GT, Gilbert JS, Labouvie E: Guided and unguided self-help for binge eating. Behav Res Ther 2000;38:259–272.

86 Stice E: Sociocultural influences on body image and eating disturbance; in Fairburn CG, Brownell KD (eds): Eating Disorders and Obesity. New York, Guilford Press, 2002, pp 103–107.

87 Spitzer RL, Yanovski S, Wadden T, Wing R, Marcus MD, Stunkard A, Devlin M, Mitchell J, Hasin D, Horne RL: Binge eating disorder: Its further validation in a multisite study. Int J Eat Disord 1993;13:137–153.

88   Wilson GT, Nonas C, Rosenblum GD: Assessment of binge eating in obese patients. Int J Eat Disord 1993;13:25–34.
89   Hay P, Fairburn CG: The validity of the DSM-IV scheme for classifying bulimic eating disorders. Int J Eat Disord 1998;23:7–15.
90   Striegel-Moore RH, Wilson GT, Wilfley DE, Elder KA, Brownell KD: Binge eating in an obese community sample. Int J Eat Disord 1998;23:27–37.
91   Telch CF, Stice E: Psychiatric comorbidity in women with binge eating disorder: Prevalence rates from a non-treatment-seeking sample. J Consult Clin Psychol 1998;66:768–776.
92   Hilbert A, Tuschen-Caffier B: Body-related cognitions in binge eating disorder and bulimia nervosa; J Soc Clin Psychol, in press.
93   Pratt EM, Telch CF, Labouvie EW, Wilson GT, Agras WS: Perfectionism in women with binge eating disorder. Int J Eat Disord 2001;29:177–186.
94   Goldfein JA, Walsh BT, LaChaussee JL, Kissileff HR, Devlin MJ: Eating behavior in binge eating disorder. Int J Eat Disord 1993;14:427–431.
95   Gosnell BA, Mitchell JE, Lancaster KL, Burgard MA, Wonderlich SA, Crosby RD: Food presentation and energy intake in a feeding laboratory study of subjects with binge eating disorder. Int J Eat Disord 2001;30:441–446.
96   Vögele C, Florin I: Psychophysiological responses to food exposure: An experimental study in binge eaters. Int J Eat Disord 1997;21:147–157.
97   Crowther JH, Snaftner J, Bonifazi DZ, Shepard KL: The role of daily hassles in binge eating. Int J Eat Disord 2001;29:449–454.
98   Fairburn CG, Cooper Z, Cooper PJ: The clinical features and maintenance of bulimia nervosa; in Brownell KD, Foreyt JP (eds): Handbook of Eating Disorders: Physiology, Psychology and Treatment of Obesity, Anorexia and Bulimia. New York, Basic Books, 1986, pp 389–404.
99   Fairburn CG, Cooper Z, Shafran R: Cognitive behaviour therapy for eating disorders: A 'transdiagnostic' theory and treatment. Behav Res Ther 2003;41:509–528.
100 Devlin MJ, Goldfein JA, Dobrow I: What is this thing called BED? Current status of binge eating disorder nosology. Int J Eat Disord 2003;34:S2–S18.

Dr. Anja Hilbert
Klinische Psychologie und Psychotherapie
Fakultät für Psychologie und Sportwissenschaft
Universität Bielefeld, Postfach 10 01 31
DE–33501 Bielefeld (Germany)
Tel. +49 521 106 4490, Fax +49 521 106 89012, E-Mail anja.hilbert@uni-bielefeld.de

Munsch S, Beglinger C (eds): Obesity and Binge Eating Disorder.
Bibl Psychiatr. Basel, Karger, 2005, No 171, pp 165–179

....

The Psychological and Pharmacological Treatment of Binge Eating Disorder

An Overview

Esther Biedert

Department of Clinical Psychology and Psychotherapy,
University of Basel, Basel, Switzerland

The eating disorders bulimia nervosa (BN) and binge eating disorder (BED) share the common symptom of binge eating as well as other psychological and behavioral characteristics. Probably due to this fact, the literature and research on the treatment of BED has been influenced heavily by the BN treatment literature. Therefore, treatments that were proofed to be efficacious for BN patients (particularly cognitive behavior therapy (CBT) and interpersonal therapy (IPT)) plus dialectical behavior therapy (DBT) were modified and used in the treatment of BED. Each of these treatments targets primarily a reduction in binge eating and associated mechanisms (e.g. relationships in IPT, affect in DBT), and secondarily weight management. Beside psychotherapy, the treatment of BED comprises traditional behavioral weight loss programs, dietary treatment and pharmacotherapy. Interestingly, traditional behavioral weight loss programs and dietary treatments produced weight loss and decreased binge eating. Antidepressant medication resulted in modest reductions in binge eating compared with placebo and, in some studies, weight loss.

Uncertainty actually exists about the most effective treatment of obese BED patients. The greatest controversy exists between exponents of the disorder-specific treatments and the experts in obesity treatment. For the first ones, the primarily aim of treatment is the reduction of binge eating, increasing body image and treatment of comorbid psychological disorders. The latter primarily have the aim of achieving weight loss. Regarding the coexistence of several etiological and maintaining factors of BED, it becomes obvious that different aspects of the disorder are relevant for treatment and that they can be targeted with different priorities. The question for the most effective intervention has not yet been definitively answered. This is also true for the individual differentiated assignment of BED patients to one specific treatment according to relevant predictors of treatment outcome.

The following gives a review about empirical studies for the treatment of BED, implicating psychotherapeutic treatment approaches with their specific contents, behavioral weight loss programs as well as treatment studies with pharmacotherapy. After the review of the available evidence, future directions for the research and treatment of BED will be discussed.

Psychological Treatment of BED

Cognitive Behavioral Therapy (CBT – Therapist-Led)
CBT for BED was modified by Fairburn et al. [1] according to the treatment of BN. CBT treatment approach of BED focuses on the eating disturbance and the associated problematic cognitions and attitudes toward eating, body shape, and weight. Food intake should be neither over- nor under-restrictive and the treatment focuses on a regular food intake with three principal meals and two to three snacks per day. Furthermore, the reduction of the intensity, duration and frequency of the binges is emphasised. The most central cognitive-behavioral techniques include self-monitoring, stimulus control, nutritional rehabilitation, problem solving, cognitive restructuring, and relapse prevention. Physical activity should be increased during treatment. The primary goal in CBT is the control of binge eating, which for many researchers is necessary before obese persons can lose weight. That is, efforts to reduce weight should be postponed until binge eating is controlled.

Several studies have shown the effectiveness of CBT for significantly reducing binge eating and decreasing depressive symptoms and negative body image [2, 3]. Reduction rates of binges differ clearly between less than 50% up to more than 90% [4, 5]. The mean abstinence rate of binges resulted between 41 and 66%, although a significant reduction in the number of binges after therapy [6–8]. These positive treatment results, significant reduction in number of binges and moderate abstinence of binges, decreased after treatment but compared to the condition before therapy there still resulted a significant long-term improvement [4, 7, 9]. Extending treatment duration enhanced the achievement rate of CBT [8]: after 12 weekly treatment sessions, achievement rate was 50%, whereas after 24 weekly sessions the rate was 66.7%. Also Fichter et al. [10] found after a CBT treatment of BED significant improvements of binges during treatment, a small but not significant worsening during the first 3 years after treatment, and again an improvement and stabilization after 4, 5 and 6 years. Six years after treatment completion, only 5.9% were suffering from BED, 7.4% suffered from BN and 7.4 showed another eating disorder. Simultaneous to the improvement of the core symptom of BED, there was also a significant reduction in depression, anxiety, somatization and other psychological symptoms [10].

Unfortunately, CBT is quite ineffective for weight loss in obese BED individuals, but BED patients who are abstinent from binge eating at the end of treatment are most likely to maintain their weight reduction at the 12- to 18-month follow-up [6, 7]. In a recent study comparing cognitive therapy (CT) with behavioral therapy (BT) in the reduction of binge eating and weight loss in BED and non-BED obese subjects, Nauta et al. [11] found different results of these two treatment conditions for binge versus weight reduction. CT was more effective than BT in terms of abstinence from binge eating at the 6-month follow-up (86 vs. 44%), but BT resulted in greater weight loss than CT at the same time point (-2.4 vs. $+0.1$ kg). Furthermore, subjects diagnosed with BED at pretreatment were more likely to show weight gain at follow-up than non-BED individuals.

Several authors refer to CBT as the BED treatment of first choice [12–17]. Although such promising results, other treatment approaches seem to be as effective as CBT [5, 9, 18].

Cognitive Behavioral Therapy (CBT – Self-Help)

Self-help approaches in generally provide several advantages over traditional therapist-led treatments because they are less expensive and easily disseminated. Also for BED individuals cognitive-behavioral techniques can be delivered effectively using self-help formats. Fairburn [19] developed a self-help manual including cognitive-behavioral techniques (e.g. self-monitoring, stimulus control, problem solving, cognitive restructuring). Carter and Fairburn [14] compared in a controlled effectiveness study a pure self-help condition with a partial self-help (some sessions were guided by a paraprofessional) condition. At the end of treatment, both treatment conditions were significantly better than the waiting-list control group and the abstinence rates were 43% for the pure self-help and 50% for the partial self-help condition. At the 6-month follow-up these improvements in reducing binge eating could be maintained.

Wells et al. [20] could confirm these abstinence rates using the same self-help manual with biweekly telephone guidance, whereas these findings are limited by an uncontrolled study design. Peterson et al. [15] evaluated three different self-help approaches in a group format: therapist led, partial self-help, and pure self-help. These types of groups were all compared with a waiting-list control group. There were no differences between the three self-help conditions concerning binge eating or abstinence rates. All three treatment groups were significantly superior to the waiting-list control group. Also for the 6- and 12-month follow-up the three self-help approaches resulted in significantly better improvements than the waiting-list condition [17]. Ghaderi et al. [21] compared the efficacy of self-help without and with guidance (pure vs. guided self-help) for patients with BN and BED using the cognitive behavioral self-help manual of Fairburn [19]. The results indicate that both forms of self-help approaches have a modest effect on the eating pathology also at the 6-month follow-up. Methodologically, these findings should be interpreted cautiously concerning the heterogeneity of the diagnostic groups and the lack of a control group.

Interpersonal Therapy (IPT)

Klerman et al. [22] developed the interpersonal therapy (IPT) for the treatment of depression. Furthermore, Fairburn et al. [23] adapted IPT for the treatment of individuals with BN. In a next step, Wilfley et al. [5] again modified the IPT for the treatment of BED following the precedent one of BN. IPT has been examined as an alternative treatment to target binge eating by directly addressing the social and interpersonal deficits observed among these individuals. Binges follow interpersonal conflicts and the resultant negative mood. Handling these interpersonal problems corresponds to the main impact factor of the treatment, which leads indirectly to the reduction of binges; hence, a strong correlation between negative mood, low self-esteem, interpersonal relationships and eating behavior is assumed [23].

The IPT treatment approach produces a clinically significant reduction in binge eating: Wilfley et al. [5] randomized 56 nonpurging bulimic individuals to either CBT or IPT. Both treatments were more effective than a waiting-list control condition in reducing the number of binge days at the end of treatment, although both treatments were associated with significant increases in binge eating at the 1-year follow-up. The rates of abstinence for at least 1 week at the 12-month follow-up were comparable between the two conditions (CBT = 46%, IPT = 40%), but neither resulted in significant weight loss. In a larger replication of this randomized study, Wilfley et al. [9] found that binge eating rates were reduced significantly after 20 weeks of either CBT or IPT and that the two treatments were comparable in efficacy. Again binge eating rates increased at the 1-year follow-up, but 59% of CBT subjects and 62% of IPT subjects remained abstinent. Furthermore, abstinence from binge eating in either treatment condition enhanced long-term weight loss, which did not differ between the two treatments at the 12-month follow-up.

Agras et al. [6] studied a sample of BED patients who were not successfully treated for their BED after CBT, but also after an additional IPT the core symptoms of BED did not get better.

Dialectical Behavior Therapy (DBT)

Telch et al. [24] adopted dialectical behavior therapy (DBT) for binge eating disorder. A considerable amount of research evidence supporting the affect regulation model of binge eating exists (for review, see Polivy and Herman [25]). Because binge eating may serve as a way to cope with underlying affective conditions, the DBT treatment model postulates that binge eating serves to regulate affect. DBT, a treatment found to be effective for borderline personality disorder [26], specifically targets emotion regulation by teaching adaptive skills to enhance emotion regulation capabilities.

So far, two studies examined the efficacy of DBT for women with BED: In an uncontrolled study, Telch et al. [27] found that a 20-week trial of DBT resulted in a substantial reduction in binge eating and an 82% binge eating abstinence rate at post-treatment. At the 6-month follow-up, the abstinence rate decreased to 70% at the 6-month follow-up and the average weight loss for subjects at the same time point was 3.9 kg. In a controlled replication of this study, Telch et al. [24] found that DBT was more effective than a waiting-list control condition in the reduction of binge eating and produced an abstinence rate of 89% at the end of treatment, which decreased to 56% at the 6-month follow-up. DBT showed at least modest weight loss (2.5 kg) at the end of treatment. Weight loss was not examined at follow-up. Compared to no treatment, the group DBT is better in eliminating binge eating [24], but unfortunately the comparison to any other treatment condition is so far outstanding.

Behavioral Weight Loss Programs – Dietary Treatment of BED

Behavioral weight loss programs to BED treatment emphasis primary on weight reduction. The reduction of binge eating is neither an explicit nor an implicit aim of treatment. These behavioral weight loss programs only limit calorie intake and increase physical activity, both on the bias of behavioral strategies. Interestingly, despite this unspecific emphasis concerning binge eating, traditional behavioral weight loss programs have been effective in reducing binges in BED individuals [28–30].

Besides the reduction in binge eating these treatment approaches cause also moderate weight loss [30–33]. This seems particularly to be so in BED individuals with moderate binge eating pathology [34]. Marcus et al. [29] and Porzelius et al. [34] could show that BED individuals lose more weight in behavioral weight loss programs than with CBT or IPT. Women with BED could reduce their weight in a behavioral weight loss program but didn't change their weight with CBT [29]. One year after completion of treatment the women in the behavioral weight loss program regained their weight; the ones in the CBT condition didn't change their weight again. A study by Goodrick et al. [31] could confirm the first part of this result, but the BED individuals in the CBT condition even had increases in their weight during treatment. Nauta et al. [11] also achieved increasing weight with CT (cognitive therapy), not only for the end of treatment but also for the 6-month follow-up.

A specific type of behavioral weight loss programs is very low calorie diet programs (VLCD), which are characterized with a significant reduction in the daily calorie intake (about 800 kcal/day). VLCDs are conducted under medical supervision and are accompanied by comprehensive weight management programs, including behavioral interventions and nutritional education [35]. Recent studies have examined the effect of VLCDs on BED individuals and they show a significant weight loss (17.5 kg by the end of treatment) as well as a significant reduction in binge eating [36, 37]. But the obvious weight loss resulted at the 12-month follow-up in a weight increase about 75%. Both studies report a significant impact of VLCDs on binge eating, that means 57% and 33% of BED individuals no longer met the diagnostic criteria at the 6- [37] and 12-month follow-ups [36], respectively.

Comparable with traditional behavioral weight loss programs, the VLCDs also have a significant impact on binge eating behavior, in spite of the absence of any specific intervention targeting binge eating. And concerning weight loss, BED subjects do as well in the VLCD programs as non-BED subjects [36, 37].

The effectiveness of behavioral weight loss programs and VLCDs is surprising, considering that such treatment approaches do not focus on the core symptom of BED, namely, the binges. These results are encouraging because with these programs two goals in the treatment of obese BED subjects can be achieved: reduction of binges and of body weight.

Overall, a variety of different psychological treatments of BED inclusive of behavioral weight loss programs appear to be comparably effective in reducing binge eating. CBT and IPT achieved similar short-term and long-term results in the treatment of BED [5, 9]. Behavioral weight loss programs turned out in the short-term to be as effective as CBT for BED [28–30]. It should be noted that 6- and 12-month follow-ups showed that CBT was superior to the behavioral weight loss program concerning the abstinence of binge eating [38]. Other therapies which have been shown to be effective in treating BED are DBT [24, 27] and guided self-help based on CBT principles [14].

These results raise some questions about treatment specificity, e.g. CBT was equal to IPT in enhancing interpersonal functioning, although CBT did not target interpersonal behavior. Similarly, IPT was equal to CBT in reductions in dietary restraint at long-term follow-up, even though the topic of dietary restraint is not targeted in IPT [9]. The reduction in binge eating obtained with different psychological treatment approaches is either consistent with a non-specific treatment effect or the distinctive therapies affect some common factor of BED.

The above-mentioned psychological approaches to BED treatment display reduced binge eating, but they show relatively minimal effects on weight loss in the long-term. There seem to be no relevant differences between psychological treatment approaches concerning weight loss. Only one study found a behavioral treatment approach superior to cognitive therapy concerning weight loss [11].

How can these minimal effects on weight loss be explained, considering that the binges are successfully reduced and thus energy intake should be decreased? One possible explanation is that energy intake during binges may be distributed to the non-binge-eating caloric intake.

Regardless of the treatment approach, the long-term abstinence of binge eating turned out to be the most predictive variable for long-term weight loss [9]. For an overview in table form of the currently existing BED treatment evaluations refer to Wonderlich et al. [39].

The conclusions to the psychological treatment approaches imply several limitations: First, the study results are hard to generalize on both sexes because most studies include women and the comparability of the studies is rather small. Even though there has been a lot of work in the field of BED on its understanding and treatment in the last years, several methodological questions remain unanswered: even in controlled studies different instruments are used to assess binge eating behavior and its associated symptoms. Furthermore, in most studies individuals with several forms of psychopathology were excluded. Thus, the results may not be generalized to BED with these forms of comorbid psychopathology, such as depressive disorders or personality disorder. Although several BED treatment approaches were evaluated, most studies compare two treatment conditions. So far no controlled evaluation exists that compares all of the above-mentioned treatment approaches including the control group. Such a study would implicate a multicenter procedure with optimal standardization of recruitment, verification of diagnostic criteria, assessment, and implementation of treatment.

Pharmacologic Treatment of BED

At present there is no established psychopharmacologic treatment for BED. There are less controlled studies of pharmacologic treatment of BED compared with controlled trials for BN. Currently, three main classes of drugs have been studied in double-blind, placebo-controlled trials in BED: antidepressants, centrally acting anti-obesity agents, and anticonvulsants. Using these three categories of medications for the treatment of BED individuals is based on different theoretical rationales: the fact that BED subjects have a high lifetime prevalence of major depressive disorder [40] provides the theoretical basis for the use of antidepressants in the treatment of BED individuals. The second line of evidence is that antidepressants have been shown to be effective in the treatment of BN [41], which has common features with BED. For the use of centrally acting appetite suppressants, the association of BED with overweight and obesity offers the theoretical background. Additionally, binge eating is associated with increased appetite and reduced satiety and some anti-obesity drugs reduce appetite, increase satiety, and induce weight loss [42, 43]. Because anticonvulsants have been successfully used in the treatment of bipolar and impulse control disorders [44, 45] and the comorbidity of BED with bipolar and impulse control disorders, the use of anticonvulsants in the treatment of BED is of interest. Additionally, some anticonvulsants have been associated with weight loss in epilepsy patients [46]. In the following, the three categories of medications and their effectiveness for the treatment of BED will be reviewed.

Antidepressants

The most studied group of antidepressants agents for the treatment of BED are selective serotonin reuptake inhibitors (SSRIs). Thus, placebo-controlled studies with fluoxetine, fluvoxamine, sertraline and citalopram have been shown to modestly but significantly reduce binge eating frequency and body weight in BED over the short term [47–50]. Controlled studies have also found the tricyclic antidepressants desipramine and imipramine to be superior to placebo in subjects with nonpurging BN and obese binge eaters [51, 52].

Malhotra et al. [53] evaluated in an open trial (nonrandomized, unblinded and uncontrolled) the effectiveness of the novel antidepressant venlafaxine. The drug blocks the reuptake of norepinephrine as well as serotonin [54]. Thus, venlafaxine has different attributes in common with other drugs: it shares the serotonin reuptake blocking properties of SSRIs, the norepinephrine reuptake blocking properties of tricyclic antidepressants, and the serotonin-norepinephrine reuptake blocking properties of the anti-obesity drug sibutramine [53]. Venlafaxine treatment resulted in significant reductions of binge-eating frequency, severity of binge eating and mood symptoms, weight, BMI, waist circumference and diastolic blood pressure [53]. These positive results are preliminary due to the naturalistic and open label venlafaxine treatment and should be confirmed with controlled trials.

Centrally Acting Appetite Suppressants

The first anti-obesity medication evaluated for the treatment of BED was dexfenfluramine [55], which was superior to placebo in reducing binge frequency. But because of its association with cardiac valve lesions dexfenfluramine is currently withdrawn from the market.

Although antidepressants are the pharmacological agents most often studied in the treatment of BED, preliminary results from an open trial suggests that the anti-obesity agent sibutramine may also be effective in reducing binge eating behavior and body weight in BED associated with obesity [56]. Sibutramine is a serotonin and norepinephrine reuptake inhibitor for the treatment of obesity. Its efficacy in initial weight loss and weight maintenance is well proved in short- and long-term clinical trials [57–60]. The drug induces weight loss by affecting the physiological process of satiety and stimulating thermogenesis [57]. On the bias of the preliminary evidence of the open trial, Appolinario et al. [61] conducted subsequently a randomized placebo-controlled trial to evaluate the efficacy and tolerability of sibutramine in obese individuals with BED. Sibutramine turned out to significantly reduce the number of binge days, which was associated with a significant weight loss and reduction in depressive symptoms. Thus, the authors conclude that sibutramine is effective in the treatment of obese individuals with BED by positively affecting main domains of the eating disorder, namely binge eating, weight and depressive symptoms.

Anticonvulsants

The most extensively studied anticonvulsant in BED is topiramate. Two open trials with obese BED patients report at least moderate reduction in frequency of binges [45, 62] and weight [62]. Recently a subsequent randomized, placebo-controlled trial [63] with the anticonvulsant topiramate replicated the earlier findings: compared with placebo, topiramate was associated with a significant reduction of frequency of binges, body mass index, weight and clinical global impression [63].

The novel antiepileptic drug zonisamide is associated with weight loss. Thus, McElroy et al. [64] preliminarily assessed in an open-label, prospective trial zonisamide in the treatment of BED. Zonisamide was effective in reducing binge-eating frequency, weight, and severity of illness. Further placebo-controlled trials will show whether these preliminary positive results can be replicated.

For an overview in table form of the currently existing evaluations of pharmacologic treatment of BED is to refer to Carter et al. [65].

Controlled and uncontrolled studies of BED pharmacotherapy indicate that a range of different medications might be effective in the treatment of BED. Despite these preliminary promising results there are some limitations to take into account. There are no long-term data on the efficacy of any drug in BED patients because all trails range only from 6 to 14 weeks' duration. Another critical point is the high response on placebo in BED patients. However, this is not exclusive to BED concerning high placebo response in clinical trials in anxiety disorders and major depression [66–69]. Furthermore, the exclusion of individuals with psychiatric comorbidity minimizes the generalization of the findings because obese BED patients have usually associated comorbid conditions. The fact that in some studies BED patients received other treatments (e.g. behavioral dietary counselling, psychotherapy) makes the attribution of the reduction of binge eating and/or weight difficult.

At last, the mechanism of action of pharmacological agents on BED is so far unknown [46] and still has to be evaluated.

Combination of Psychotherapy and Pharmacotherapy

The most added and studied medications in a combined treatment approach for BED are antidepressants [28, 52, 70–72], and psychotherapy consists of CBT with or without behavioral weight loss. CBT resulted superior to drug treatment alone [70–72] and in almost all trials medication did not add to the efficacy of CBT in reducing binge eating frequency [28, 70–72]. Agras et al. [28] could show that antidepressant medication can enhance weight loss beyond the effects of CBT and behavioral weight loss.

In a randomized, double-blind, placebo-controlled study, Bauer et al. [73] assessed the effect of sibutramine in obese subjects with and without subclinical BED. Subjects were randomly assigned to 16 weeks' treatment with either sibutramine or placebo while simultaneously participating in a cognitive-behavioral group weight loss program. Sibutramine combined with the weight loss program increased weight loss in subjects with and without subclinical BED compared to the weight loss program alone. Concerning the binges, only the behavioral weight loss program but not sibutramine improved binge eating frequency and eating-related psychopathology [73].

Conclusions

Psychological (CBT, IPT, DBT) and dietary approaches to BED treatment show reasonable efficacy in reducing binge eating, but limited to moderate efficacy in weight loss. The mentioned treatment approaches are effective for about 50–60% of BED patients [74]. CBT proved to be effective in reducing binge eating frequency and intensity and associated symptoms. The treatment efficacy of IPT is similar to that of CBT. Preliminary results of the DBT treatment approach also show it to be an effective treatment possibility for BED patients in enhancing eating psychopathology. Behavioral weight loss programs reduced binge eating behavior and weight; however, the long-term maintenance of the achieved weight loss is mostly bad. Behavioral weight loss programs have two advantages over

CBT and IPT concerning the significant weight loss (at least in the short term) and it is easier to disseminate because it does not require the same training and expertise and is so implementable by different health care professionals.

The fact that different psychological treatment approaches with different content and emphasis are effective in treating BED patients raises the question about specific and non-specific treatment effects and about predictors of treatment outcome. Despite the findings on the apparent non-specificity of treatment response in BED, it would be too early to conclude that all BED patients respond equally well to all treatment approaches [75] because non-specific influences should be controlled in further studies. So far, the results concerning predictors of outcome in obese BED patients are heterogeneous. Variables that resulted significant in one study could not be replicated in others. But there is a homogenous result for a negative predictive value of the treatment outcome for the age of onset of BED [6, 8], the severity of binge eating [4, 6, 7], number of binges before treatment [16], and reduced self-efficacy [76, 77]. These findings let us assume that the longer and more chronic the eating pathology, the more difficult is its successful treatment. Unanswered are questions about predictive variables in connection with obesity (e.g. age of onset of obesity, number of diets, weight before treatment).

For the pharmacological treatment of BED there are actually three classes of agents that are potentially usable: antidepressants, anti-obesity medications, and anticonvulsants. Currently, antidepressants, and within this class the SSRIs, are the most studied drugs for BED treatment. SSRIs are shown to modestly reduce binge eating and weight. The anti-obesity medication sibutramine turned out to be also effective in decreasing binge eating behavior and weight. The same resulted from the evaluation of topiramate and zonisamide, both novel anticonvulsants. All this medications seem to be associated with positive effects on binge eating and weight in BED patients; however, questions about the optimal duration of treatment, the long-term maintenance of effects after cessation of drugs, optimal medication selection, dosing, and the efficacy of combined treatment approaches to BED (psychotherapy and pharmacotherapy) are still unanswered. More and larger randomized and controlled trials are needed for further evaluation and comparison of the effects of the different medications.

BED seems to be quite a reactive disorder that remits spontaneously without clinical attention and has a strong placebo response rate. But the latter is not specific to BED. Two studies with community samples show that without treatment partial remissions of BED of 48% and 90%, respectively, after 6 months [78] no longer met the criteria at the 5-year follow-up [79]. Carter et al. [14] found a 34% reduction in binge eating during a 3 months' waiting list control condition. And even if the mentioned drugs are effective for the treatment of BED, the strong placebo responses suggest a conservative use of medications in BED: placebo response rates for BED are high across all the three main classes of drugs [47]; i.e. 46% [50, 63]. As cited in Stunkard and Allison [80], many trials with pharmacotherapy, independent of the diagnostic categories, use a 50% reduction in symptoms as criterion of responder status. Concerning this criterion, placebo responses in the treatment of BED are close to an effective treatment. The strong placebo responsiveness and the modest weight loss question the value of pharmacotherapy in the treatment of BED [80] or at least argue for a conservative use when administered alone.

Actually, there are several effective possibilities to treat obese patients with BED although not all mentioned treatment approaches have the same status of evaluation and some findings are still preliminary. Further controlled research in both domains, psychotherapy and pharmacotherapy, is needed to find out effective treatment approaches. Particularly more research about outcome predictors is required to direct individual patients toward the most efficacious treatment approaches. This concerns BED in the adult population, but there are also open questions concerning BED in children and adolescents [81]. For further reading about BED in childhood see the chapter by Munsch and Hilbert in this volume [pp. 180–196].

References

1   Fairburn CG, Marcus MD, Wilson GT: Cognitive behaviour therapy for binge eating and bulimia nervosa: A comprehensive treatment manual; in Fairburn CG, Wilson GT (eds): Binge Eating: Nature, Assessment and Treatment. New York, Guilford Press, 1993, pp 361–404.
2   Wilfley DE, Cohen LR: Psychological treatment of bulimia nervosa and binge eating disorder. Psychopharmacol Bull 1997;33:437–454.
3   Williamson DA, Martin CK: Binge eating disorder: A review of the literature after publication of DSM-IV. Eat Weight Disord 1999;4:103–114.
4   Telch CF, Agras WS, Rossiter EM, Wilfley D, Kenardy J: Group cognitive-behavioral treatment for the nonpurging bulimic: An initial evaluation. J Consult Clin Psychol 1990;58:629–635.
5   Wilfley DE, Agras WS, Telch CF, Rossiter EM, Schneider JA, Cole AG, Sifford LA, Raeburn SD: Group cognitive-behavioral therapy and group interpersonal psychotherapy for the nonpurging bulimic individual: A controlled comparison. J Consult Clin Psychol 1993;61:296–305.
6   Agras WS, Telch CF, Arnow B, Eldredge K, Detzer MJ, Henderson J, Marnell M: Does interpersonal therapy help patients with binge eating disorder who fail to respond to cognitive-behavioral therapy? J Consult Clin Psychol 1995;63:356–360.
7   Agras WS, Telch CF, Arnow B, Eldredge K, Marnell M: One-year follow-up of cognitive-behavioral therapy for obese individuals with binge eating disorder. J Consult Clin Psychol 1997;65:343–347.
8   Eldredge KL, Stewart Agras W, Arnow B, Telch CF, Bell S, Castonguay L, Marnell M: The effects of extending cognitive-behavioral therapy for binge eating disorder among initial treatment nonresponders. Int J Eat Disord 1997;21:347–352.
9   Wilfley DE, Welch RR, Stein RI, Spurrell EB, Cohen LR, Saelens BE, Dounchis JZ, Frank MA, Wiseman CV, Matt GE: A randomized comparison of group cognitive-behavioral therapy and group interpersonal psychotherapy for the treatment of overweight individuals with binge-eating disorder. Arch Gen Psychiatry 2002;59:713–721.

10   Fichter MM, Quadflieg N, Gnutzmann A: Binge eating disorder: Treatment outcome over a 6-year course. J Psychosom Res 1998;44:385–405.

11   Nauta H, Hospers H, Kok G, Jansen A: A comparison between a cognitive and a behavioral treatment for obese binge eaters and obese non-binge eaters. Behav Ther 2000;31:441–461.

12   Ricca V, Mannucci E, Zucchi T, Rotella CM, Faravelli C: Cognitive-behavioural therapy for bulimia nervosa and binge eating disorder: A review. Psychother Psychosom 2000;69: 287–295.

13   Loeb KL, Wilson GT, Gilbert JS, Labouvie E: Guided and unguided self-help for binge eating. Behav Res Ther 2000;38:259–272.

14   Carter JC, Fairburn CG: Cognitive-behavioral self-help for binge eating disorder: A controlled effectiveness study. J Consult Clin Psychol 1998;66:616–623.

15   Peterson CB, Mitchell JE, Engbloom S, Nugent S, Mussell MP, Miller JP: Group cognitive-behavioral treatment of binge eating disorder: A comparison of therapist-led versus self-help formats. Int J Eat Disord 1998;24:125–136.

16   Peterson CB, Crow SJ, Nugent S, Mitchell JE, Engbloom S, Mussell MP: Predictors of treatment outcome for binge eating disorder. Int J Eat Disord 2000;28:131–138.

17   Peterson CB, Mitchell JE, Engbloom S, Nugent S, Pederson Mussell M, Crow SJ, Thuras P: Self-help versus therapist-led group cognitive-behavioral treatment of binge eating disorder at follow-up. Int J Eat Disord 2001;30:363–374.

18   Wilfley DE: Paper presented at the Eating Disorders Research Society. San Diego, 1999.

19   Fairburn CG: Overcoming Binge Eating. New York, Guilford Press, 1995.

20   Wells AM, Garvin V, Dohm FA, Striegel-Moore RH: Telephone-based guided self-help for binge eating disorder: A feasibility study. Int J Eat Disord 1997;21:341–346.

21   Ghaderi A, Scott B: Pure and guided self-help for full and sub-threshold bulimia nervosa and binge eating disorder. Br J Clin Psychol 2003;42:257–269.

22   Klerman GL, Weissman MM, Rounsaville BJ, Chevron ES: Interpersonal Psychotherapy of Depression. New York, Basic Books, 1984.

23   Fairburn CG, Jones R, Peveler RC, Carr SJ, Solomon RA, O'Connor ME, Burton J, Hope RA: Three psychological treatments for bulimia nervosa: A comparative trial. Arch Gen Psychiatry 1991;48:463–469.

24   Telch CF, Agras WS, Linehan MM: Dialectical behavior therapy for binge eating disorder. J Consult Clin Psychol 2001;69:1061–1065.

25   Polivy J, Herman CP: Etiology of binge eating: Psychological mechanisms; in Fairburn CG, Wilson GT (eds): Binge Eating: Nature, Assessment, and Treatment. New York, Guilford Press, 1993, pp 173–205.

26   Linehan M: Cognitive-Behavioral treatment of Borderline Personality Disorder. New York, Guilford Press, 1993.

27   Telch CF, Agras WS, Linehan MM: Group dialectical behavior therapy for Binge Eating Disorder: A preliminary uncontrolled trial. Assoc Adv Behav Ther 2000;31:569–582.

28   Agras WS, Telch CF, Arnow B, Eldredge K, Wilfley DE, Raeburn SD, Henderson J, Marnell M: Weight loss, cognitive-behavioral desipramine treatments in binge eating disorder: An additive design. Behav Ther 1994;25:209–238.

29   Marcus MD, Wing RR, Fairburn CG: Cognitive behavioral treatment of binge eating versus behavioral weight control in the treatment of binge eating disorder. Ann Behav Med 1995; 17: S090.

30   Gladis MM, Wadden TA, Vogt R, Foster G, Kuehnel RH, Bartlett SJ: Behavioral treatment of obese binge eaters: Do they need different care? J Psychosom Res 1998;44:375–384.

31   Goodrick GK, Walker CC, Poston WW, Kimball KT, Reeves RS, Foreyt JP: Nondieting versus dieting treatment for overweight binge eating-women. J Consult Clin Psychol 1999;2:363–368.

32   Sherwood NE, Jeffery RW, Wing RR: Binge status as a predictor of weight loss treatment outcome. Int J Obes Relat Metab Disord 1999;23:485–493.

33   Wilson GT, Fairburn CG: The treatment of binge eating disorder (special section). Eur Eat Disord Rev 2000;8:351–354.

34   Porzelius LK, Houston C, Smith M, Arfken C, Fisher E: Comparison of a standard behavioral weight loss treatment and a binge eating weight loss treatment. Behav Ther 1995;26:119–134.

35 Wadden TA, Bartlett SJ: Very low calorie diets: An overview and appraisal; in Wadden TA, VanItallie TB (eds): Treatment of the Seriously Obese Patients. New York, Guilford Press, 1992, pp 440–479.

36 de Zwaan M, Mitchell JE, Mussell MP, Raymond NC, Seim HC, Specker SM, Crosby RD: Short-term cognitive-behavioral treatment does not improve outcome on a comprehensive very-low-calorie diet program in obese women with binge eating disorder. 2003;in press.

37 Raymond NC, de Zwaan M, Mitchell JE, Ackard D, Thuras P: Effect of a very low calorie diet on the diagnostic category of individuals with binge eating disorder. Int J Eat Disord 2002;31:49–56.

38 Nauta H, Hospers H, Jansen A: One-year follow-up effects of two obesity treatments on psychological well-being and weight. Br J Hlth Psychol 2001;6:271–284.

39 Wonderlich SA, de Zwaan M, Mitchell JE, Peterson C, Crow S: Psychological and dietary treatments of binge eating disorder: Conceptual implications. Int J Eat Disord 2003;34(suppl):S58–S73.

40 Yanovski SZ, Nelson JE, Dubbert BK, Spitzer RL: Association of binge eating disorder and psychiatric comorbidity in obese subjects. Am J Psychiatry 1993;150:1472–1479.

41 Hudson JI, Pope HG Jr, Carter WP: Pharmacologic therapy of bulimia nervosa; in Goldstein D (ed): The Management of Eating Disorders and Obesity. Totowa, Humana Press, 1999, pp 19–32.

42 Rothman RB, Baumann MH: Therapeutic and adverse actions of serotonin transporter substrates. Pharmacol Ther 2002;95:73–88.

43 Guss JL, Kissileff HR, Devlin MJ, Zimmerli E, Walsh BT: Binge size increases with body mass index in women with binge-eating disorder. Obes Res 2002;10:1021–1029.

44 Krüger S, Kennedy SH: Psychopharmacotherapy of anorexia nervosa, bulimia nervosa and binge eating disorder (review). J Psychiatr Neurosci 2000;25:497–508.

45 Shapira NA, Goldsmith TD, McElroy SL: Treatment of binge-eating disorder with topiramate: A clinical case series. J Clin Psychiatry 2000;61:368–372.

46 Appolinarion JC, McElroy SL: Pharmacological approaches in the treatment of binge eating disorder. Curr Drug Targets 2004;5:301–307.

47 Hudson JI, McElroy SL, Raymond NC, Crow S, Keck PE Jr, Carter WP, Mitchell JE, Strakowski SM, Pope HG Jr, Coleman BS, Jonas JM: Fluvoxamine in the treatment of binge-eating disorder: A multicenter placebo-controlled, double-blind trial. Am J Psychiatry 1998;155:1756–1762.

48 Mayer LE, Walsh BT: The use of selective serotonin reuptake inhibitors in eating disorders. J Clin Psychiatry 1998;59(suppl 15):28–34.

49 Arnold LM, McElroy SL, Hudson JI, Welge JA, Bennett AJ, Keck PE: A placebo-controlled, randomized trial of fluoxetine in the treatment of binge-eating disorder. J Clin Psychiatry 2002; 63:1028–1033.

50 McElroy SL, Casuto LS, Nelson EB, Lake KA, Soutullo CA, Keck PE Jr, Hudson JI: Placebo-controlled trial of sertraline in the treatment of binge eating disorder. Am J Psychiatry 2000; 157:1004–1006.

51 McCann UD, Agras WS: Successful treatment of nonpurging bulimia nervosa with desipramine: A double-blind, placebo-controlled study. Am J Psychiatry 1990;147:1509–1513.

52 Laederach-Hofmann K, Graf C, Horber F, Lippuner K, Lederer S, Michel R, Schneider M: Imipramine and diet counseling with psychological support in the treatment of obese binge eaters: A randomized, placebo-controlled double-blind study. Int J Eat Disord 1999;26:231–244.

53 Malhotra S, King KH, Welge JA, Brusman-Lovins L, McElroy SL: Venlafaxine treatment of binge-eating disorder associated with obesity: A series of 35 patients. J Clin Psychiatry 2002;63:802–806.

54 Harvey AT, Rudolph RL, Preskorn SH: Evidence of the dual mechanisms of action of venlafaxine. Arch Gen Psychiatry 2000;57:503–509.

55 Stunkard A, Berkowitz R, Tanrikut C, Reiss E, Young L: d-Fenfluramine treatment of binge eating disorder. Am J Psychiatry 1996;153:1455–1459.

56 Appolinario JC, Godoy-Matos A, Fontenelle LF, Carraro L, Cabral M, Vieira A, Coutinho W: An open-label trial of sibutramine in obese patients with binge-eating disorder. J Clin Psychiatry 2002;63:28–30.

57 Yanovski SZ, Yanovski JA: Obesity. N Engl J Med 2002;346:591–602.

58 Ryan DH, Kaiser P, Bray GA: Sibutramine: A novel new agent for obesity treatment. Obes Res 1995;3(suppl 4):553S–559S.

59 Bray GA, Ryan DH, Gordon D, Heidingsfelder S, Cerise F, Wilson K: A double-blind randomized placebo-controlled trial of sibutramine. Obes Res 1996;4:263–270.

Biedert

60   James WP, Astrup A, Finer N, Hilsted J, Kopelman P, Rossner S, Saris WH, Van Gaal LF: Effect of sibutramine on weight maintenance after weight loss: A randomised trial. STORM Study Group. Sibutramine Trial of Obesity Reduction and Maintenance. Lancet 2000;356:2119–2125.

61   Appolinario JC, Bacaltchuk J, Sichieri R, Claudino AM, Godoy-Matos A, Morgan C, Zanella MT, Coutinho W: A randomized, double-blind, placebo-controlled study of sibutramine in the treatment of binge-eating disorder. Arch Gen Psychiatry 2003;60:1109–1116.

62   Appolinario JC, Fontenelle LF, Papelbaum M, Bueno JR, Coutinho W: Topiramate use in obese patients with binge eating disorder: An open study. Can J Psychiatry 2002;47:271–273.

63   McElroy SL, Arnold LM, Shapira NA, Keck PE Jr, Rosenthal NR, Karim MR, Kamin M, Hudson JI: Topiramate in the treatment of binge eating disorder associated with obesity: A randomized, placebo-controlled trial. Am J Psychiatry 2003;160:255–261.

64   McElroy SL, Kotwal R, Hudson JI, Nelson EB, Keck PE: Zonisamide in the treatment of binge-eating disorder: An open-label, prospective trial. J Clin Psychiatry 2004;65:50–56.

65   Carter WP, Hudson JI, Lalonde JK, Pindyck L, McElroy SL, Pope HG Jr: Pharmacologic treatment of binge eating disorder. Int J Eat Disord 2003;34(suppl):S74–S88.

66   Schweizer E, Rickels K: Placebo response in generalized anxiety: Its effect on the outcome of clinical trials. J Clin Psychiatry 1997;58(suppl 11):30–38.

67   Versiani M: A review of 19 double-blind placebo-controlled studies in social anxiety disorder (social phobia). World J Biol Psychiatry 2000;1:27–33.

68   Schatzberg AF, Kraemer HC: Use of placebo control groups in evaluating efficacy of treatment of unipolar major depression. Biol Psychiatry 2000;47:736–744.

69   Walsh BT, Seidman SN, Sysko R, Gould M: Placebo response in studies of major depression: Variable, substantial, and growing. JAMA 2002;287:1840–1847.

70   Devlin M: Psychotherapy and medication for binge eating disorder. International Conference on Eating Disorders, Boston, 2002.

71   Grilo CM, Masheb RM, Heninger G, Wilson GT: Psychotherapy and medication for binge eating disorder. International Conference on Eating Disorders, Boston, 2002.

72   Ricca V, Mannucci E, Mezzani B, Moretti S, Di Bernardo M, Bertelli M, Rotella CM, Faravelli C: Fluoxetine and fluvoxamine combined with individual cognitive-behaviour therapy in binge eating disorder: A one-year follow-up study. Psychother Psychosom 2001;70:298–306.

73   Bauer C, Fischer A, Keller U: Effect of sibutramine in obese subjects with subclinical binge eating disorder. Submitted, 2004.

74   Stice E: Clinical implications of psychosocial research on bulimia nervosa and binge-eating disorder. J Clin Psychol 1999;55:675–683.

75   Wilfley DE, Wilson GT, Agras WS: The clinical significance of binge eating disorder. Int J Eat Disord 2003;34(suppl):S96–S106.

76   Miller PM, Watkins JA, Sargent RG, Rickert EJ: Self-efficacy in overweight individuals with binge eating disorder. Obes Res 1999;7:552–555.

77   Goodrick GK, Pendleton VR, Kimball KT, Carlos Poston WS, Reeves RS, Foreyt JP: Binge eating severity, self-concept, dieting self-efficacy and social support during treatment of binge eating disorder. Int J Eat Disord 1999;26:295–300.

78   Cachelin FM, Striegel-Moore RH, Elder KA, Pike KM, Wilfley DE, Fairburn CG: Natural course of a community sample of women with binge eating disorder. Int J Eat Disord 1999;25:45–54.

79   Fairburn CG, Cooper Z, Doll HA, Norman P, O'Connor M: The natural course of bulimia nervosa and binge eating disorder in young women. Arch Gen Psychiatry 2000;57:659–665.

80   Stunkard AJ, Allison KC: Binge eating disorder: disorder or marker? Int J Eat Disord 2003;34(suppl):S107–S116.

81   Marcus MD, Kalarchian MA: Binge eating in children and adolescents. Int J Eat Disord 2003;34(suppl):S47–S57.

Esther Biedert, lic. phil.
University of Basel, Department of Clinical Psychology and Psychotherapy
Missionsstrasse 60/62, CH–4055 Basel (Switzerland)
Tel. +41 61 267 06 52, Fax +41 61 267 06 59, E-Mail esther.biedert@unibas.ch

Munsch S, Beglinger C (eds): Obesity and Binge Eating Disorder.
Bibl Psychiatr. Basel, Karger, 2005, No 171, pp 180–196

....

Binge Eating Disorder in Childhood – What Do We Know About It?

Simone Munsch[a], *Anja Hilbert*[b]

[a]Institut für Psychologie, Universität Basel, Basel, Schweiz; [b]Department of
Psychiatry, School of Medicine, Washington University, St. Louis, Mo., USA

The research criteria of binge eating disorder (BED) were included in the
4th edition of the Diagnostic and Statistical Manual of Mental Disorders in
1994 [1]. Increasing evidence suggests that BED is associated with significant
psychopathology and comorbidity [2]. Already children and adolescents may
suffer from the symptomatology of BED [3, 4]. In this chapter, we describe the
current state of research on symptomatology, epidemiology, etiology, and outline guidelines for the treatment of BED in childhood.

Description and Classification

Adults with BED suffer from regular binge eating episodes, during which
they typically ingest large quantities of food and experience a sense of loss of
control over eating [1]. As opposed to individuals with bulimia nervosa (BN),
individuals with BED do not engage regularly in compensatory behavior such
as purging, fasting or excessive physical activity. Eating behavior in BED is
usually chaotic and characterized by a general tendency to overeat [5–7]. Binge
eating is often triggered by emotional cues, especially negative mood [8, 9] and
may serve for affect regulation purposes, e.g. coping with negative mood states
such as anxiety [10]. In clinical samples, most BED patients are obese [11–13;
see also Tuschen-Caffier and Schlüssel, this vol., pp. 138–148].

Binge eating without regular compensatory behavior was found to occur in
children and adolescents, in clinical and population-based samples [see e.g. 3].
Loss of control over eating emerges during regular meals or special occasions

Table 1. Provisional BED research criteria for children [3]

a. Recurrent episodes of binge eating: an episode of binge eating is characterized by both of the following
  1. Food seeking in the absence of hunger (e.g. after a full meal)
  2. A sense of lack of control over eating (e.g. endorse that, 'When I start to eat, I just can't stop')
b. Binge episodes are associated with one or more of the following
  1. Food seeking in response to negative affect (e.g. sadness, boredom, restlessness)
  2. Food seeking as a reward
  3. Sneaking or hiding food
c. Symptoms persist over a period of 3 months
d. Eating is not associated with the regular use of inappropriate compensatory behaviors (e.g. purging, fasting, excessive exercise) and does not occur exclusively during the course of anorexia nervosa or bulimia nervosa

---

such as parties or restaurant visits [14]. Similar to BED in adults, a sense of loss of control, but not the amount of food intake seems to influence the subjective experience of binge eating [14]. Loss of control is further associated with greater eating disorder and general psychopathology (e.g. anxiety and depressiveness), a higher BMI and higher body fat percentage [15–19].

Despite similarities of adult and child symptomatology of BED, the DSM-IV research criteria of BED may not fully apply to children. For example it remains unclear how binge eating and especially loss of control presents, if children's access to food is usually regulated by their parents [14, 20]. Children may also show a greater fluctuation of their eating disorder symptomatology over time, therefore the time criterion (i.e. recurrent episodes of binge eating, at least 2 days a week for 6 months) may need to cover a shorter time period for the diagnosis of BED in childhood and adolescence [21]. Further, it remains unclear whether children and adolescents experience feelings of guilt, depressiveness or disgust following binge eating, as it is definitional for adult BED [1].

In other childhood onset eating disorders such as anorexia nervosa (AN) and BN, age-adapted diagnostic criteria have shown to be more reliable for classification than criteria to classify mental disorders in adults (Great Ormond Street Criteria) [22, 23]. Accordingly, Marcus and Kalarchian [2] proposed preliminary criteria for BED in childhood and adolescence younger than 14 years of age. These research criteria have not yet been validated empirically (table 1).

Epidemiology

Based on different definitions of binge eating, the prevalence of regular binge eating episodes in children and adolescents ranges from 7 to 28% [19, 24–29].

This wide variation is due to the almost exclusive assessment of regular binge eating with self-report questionnaires. In contrast to this, the prevalence of the full syndrome of BED according to the DSM-IV criteria in children and adolescents is most often assessed with interviews and amounts to 1–3% [17, 20, 29].

Until now, most research on binge eating in children and adolescents is based on self-report questionnaires. Décaluwe and Braet [30] recommend face to face clinical interviews to assess disordered eating behavior in children for further research (e.g. ChEDE, Child EDE [31]). For an overview of the prevalence of binge eating behavior and BED in childhood in different populations, see table 2.

Research about the course and outcome of binge eating and BED in the pediatric population is at a very early stage [see also Hilbert, this vol., pp. 149–164]. Although Stice et al. [32] showed a moderate stability of uncontrolled eating from birth until the age of 5 years and although in other eating disorders (AN, BN) symptoms often present in childhood as well as in adults [33–35], it is largely unknown if binge eating in childhood is continuous with BED in adulthood [3].

Assessment

The assessment and diagnosis of the symptomatology of BED is usually based on the exploration of child, parents (especially if young children are concerned), and other significant others [36, 37].

For the assessment of the symptomatology of BED in children at 9–11 years of age self-report questionnaires may be useful [36]. Structured interviews, however, likely improve reliability of diagnosis [30, 38, 39]. An advantage of structured interviews such as the ChEDE [31] for the diagnosis of childhood eating disorders is that the interviewer can provide definitions and assure understanding of complex characteristics such as binge eating or sense of loss of control. Further information about daily nutritional and eating behavior may be assessed by self-monitoring (e.g. when, what, and how much was eaten) [40].

Table 3 shows a selection of questionnaires and structured interviews for the assessment of BED symptomatology in children and adolescents, available in English and German. In addition, self-report questionnaires that have not yet been validated in German, e.g. the Children's Eating Behavior Inventory (CEBI [41]) and the Questionnaire of Eating and Weight Patterns – Adults version (QEWP-A, [42]) were frequently applied in English.

Etiology

Retrospective risk factor studies in adults with BED [43–49] suggest a range of adverse childhood experiences as for example shape and weight teasing as

Table 2. Prevalence of binge eating behavior and BED in children and adolescents

Authors	Sample characteristics (n, age, sex, mean body mass index, BMI)	Study design	Assessment methods	Definition of binge eating behavior or BED and point prevalence rates
Population-based surveys: Binge eating				
Whitaker et al. [24]	5,996 students, 14–17 years	cross-sectional	Eating Symptoms Inventory, questionnaire [24]	binge eating, loss of control over eating not defined binge eating episodes: 33% M, 7% F recurrent binges: 19% M, 6% F
Childress et al. [25]	3,175 students, 10–13 years	cross-sectional	Kids' Eating Disorders Survey, questionnaire [25]	binge eating, defined as intake of large amounts of food eaten within 2 hours binge eating: 26.3% M, 6.5% F
Ledoux et al. [80]	3,287 students, 12–19 years (1,541 males, 1,716 females)	cross-sectional, retrospective (12 months)	survey including self-report questionnaire focusing on eating behaviors [81]	binge eating, defined as eating an enormous amount of food with the fear of not being able to stop. binge eating: 20.5% M, 28.1% F binge eating episodes twice a week: 2.7% M, 3.7% F
Devaud et al. [82]	1,084 female students, 15–20 years	cross-sectional	Swiss Multicenter Adolescent Health Survey, a self-report questionnaire focusing on eating behavior [83, 84]	binge eating, not specified: 9.1% at least once a week
Field et al. [26]	26,765 students, 9–14 years	cross-sectional	Nurses' Health Study II, survey: McKnight Risk Factor Survey [85], Youth Risk Behavior Surveillance System questionnaire [86]	binge eating, not specified, at least monthly: 0.8% M, 1.9% F

Table 2 (continued)

Authors	Sample characteristics (n, age, sex, mean body mass index, BMI)	Study design	Assessment methods	Definition of binge eating behavior or BED and point prevalence rates
Croll et al. [27]	81,247 students, 14–17 years	cross-sectional, retrospective (12 months)	Minnesota Student Survey, self-report questionnaire [86–88]	binge eating, defined as eating a large amount in a short period of time with an out of control-feeling over eating. binge eating: 12.5% M, 25.6% F
Population-based surveys: bed				
Ackard et al. [17]	4,746 students, 11–18 years (2,377 males, 2,357 females)	cross-sectional	Project EAT (Eating Among Teens) survey [17], sections of adult version Questionnaire of Eating and Weight Patterns-Revised QEWP-R [89]	binge eating syndrome, defined as objective overeating, loss of control 'a few times a week' subclinical level of binge eating, defined as objective overeating and loss of control: 2.4% M, 7.9% F, every day: 0.9% M, 3.1% F overeating, defined according to QEWP-R: 7.8% M, 17.3% F
Johnson et al. [29]	822 students, 14–19 years (47.45% males, 52.55% females)[a]	cross-sectional	Questionnaire of Eating and Weight Patterns – adolescent version QEWP-A [42]	bed, defined according to QEWP-A: 1% varying degrees of subthreshold binge eating problems: 26% African-American boys, 19% white boys, 17% African-American girls, 18% white girls
Morgan et al. [14]	112 children, 6–10 years, 52 males, 60 females, BMI ≥ 85. Percentile	cross-sectional	Questionnaire of Eating and Weight Patterns – adolescent version QEWP-A [42]	bed, defined according to QEWP-A: 5.3% loss of control over eating: 33.1%

Obese treatment-seeking samples

Berkowitz et al. [90]	51 girls, 14–16 years, mean BMI 36.7	cross-sectional	diagnostic interview	manifest binge eating, not specified: 30%
Severi et al. [91]	52 obese children, 13–19 years	cross-sectional	clinical interview following DSM-IV criteria [92]	binge eating problems, not specified: 18% M, 27% F
Britz et al. [28]	47 students, 15–21 years, 17 males, 30 females, mean BMI 42.4 (clinical sample) 1,655 students, 15–21 years, 805 males, 850 females (control group)	cross-sectional	Munich-Composite International Diagnostic Interview [93]	binge eating episodes, defined as having ever experienced episodes of intake of large amounts of food with lack of control: 35% M, 57% F
Isnard et al. [19]	102 adolescents, 12–17 years, 35 males, 67 females, mean BMI 36.4 (clinical sample)	cross-sectional	Binge Eating Scale [94]	moderate to severe and severe binge eating, defined according to BES score: >18: 16%; >26: 3%
Decaluwé et al. [95]	126 children/clinical sample, 10–16 years	cross-sectional	Eating Disorder-Questionnaire EDE-Q [96],	binge eating episodes: 36.5% binge eating episodes twice a week or more often: 6%

[a] BMI only mentioned if >30.

Table 3. For children and adolescents adapted methods for the assessment of the symptomatology of BED available in an English and a German version

Instrument	Age	Design and diagnostic information	Psychometric properties	Notes
Structured interviews for eating disorders for children and adolescents				
Eating Disorder Examination for children (ChEDE [31])	age 8–14	35 items (diagnostic items and items describing eating disorder pathology); subscales restraint, eating concern, shape concern, weight concern; analysis: diagnosis, subscale and global scores	support for discriminant and convergent validity; subscale scores consistent with adult norms	adapted version of the Eating Disorder Examination [97, 98]
Self-report questionnaire for children and adolescents				
Body Image Assessment for children and preadolescents (BIA-C, BIA-P [99])	≥age 8	age- and gender-specific body image silhouettes for the assessment of negative body image; analysis: self-ideal-discrepancy	support for retest-reliability and convergent validity	
Dutch Eating Behavior Questionnaire for children (DEBQ-K [100])	age 7–13	30 items; subscales externally determined eating behavior, emotional-induced eating behavior, restrictive eating behavior; analysis: subscale scores	retest-reliability, internal consistency of subscales (Cronbach α > 0.80), factorial validity, reference norms for children ages 11 to 12[a]	childrens version of the Dutch Eating Behavior Questionnaire (DEBQ; [101])
Eating Disorder Examination-Questionnaire for adolescents (EDE-Q [102])	age 12–14	36 items; subscales restraint, eating concern, shape concern, weight concern and diagnostic items; analysis: diagnosis, subscale and global scores	reference norms for adolescents	the EDE-Q [96] is the self-report version of the Eating Disorder Examination [97, 98]

[a] Psychometric properties from nonclinical applications.

Table 4. Childhood and adolescence risk factors for binge eating

Risk factors	References
Childhood traits such as negative self-evaluation, shyness, behavioral problems, and depressive symptoms	[43]
Parental depression (ever)	[43]
Physical and sexual abuse in childhood	[43, 46]
Childhood obesity	[43, 49]
Dieting	[43, 103]
Frequent weight and shape-related teasing	[43, 47, 48]
Shape concern, modeling of disordered eating, depressive feelings, pressure to be thin, emotional eating, high BMI, low self-esteem, lack of social support	[44–46]
Familial transmission of disordered eating: Bulimic symptoms of the mother at birth, child's shape concerns, and parental overweight predict secretive eating; restrictive eating of the mother and pressure to be thin predict overeating; reinforcing processes during family meals (e.g. mother's prompting high eating rates and large bites) might be conditioned on the person of the mother as a discriminative stimulus of children's faster eating with larger bites	[32, 52, 104]
Mother's restriction of the portion size of children's meals precedes eating in the absence of hunger; the effect is modulated by the presence of childhood obesity	[51, 105, 106]
Concurrent affective disorders, especially dysthymia	[50]

well as a predisposition for depressive mood and obesity and the transmission of dysfunctional eating behavior such as dieting as etiological factors of BED (table 4). Further retrospective studies in adolescents [50] refer to a bi-directional association between binge eating and depression: on the one hand, binge eating may precede affective disorders in adolescents, and on the other hand chronically depressed mood may increase the risk for onset or recurrence of regular binge eating [50]. Prospective long-term studies investigating the association between child-feeding practices and children's eating behavior [32, 51] suggest that overeating in the absence of hunger is predicted by higher levels of the mother's attempts to restrict children's eating. Maternal attempts to control the child's intake might initiate initial overeating or binge eating episodes, which in turn, may initiate self-imposed restrictive dieting attempts in children. These findings are particularly clear for adolescent girls [51]. Laessle et al. [52] revealed in an experimental study that overweight children ate faster, with a greater bite size and accelerated eating rate only when the mother was present. This finding underlines the role of specific social stimulus conditions as a trigger of excessive caloric intake [52–54]. Emerging genetic epidemiological

Table 5. Hypothetical protocol for the treatment of BED in childhood and adolescence

Goals	Interventions	
	children	parents
Initial treatment phase		
Motivational phase treatment rationale	psychoeducation on the etiology and maintenance of obesity socratic dialog about pros and contras of the treatment	psychoeducation on the etiology and maintenance of obesity pro and contra of the parent's role as children's trainers
Symptom management coping with antecedents of uncontrolled and binge eating	self-monitoring and analysis of binge situations, stimulus control (nutritional management), response prevention, self-reinforcement training	supervising and reinforcement of children's efforts of coping with binge situations, motivational techniques (e.g. reinforcement plans)
Social competence training assertiveness training, coping with teasing	assertiveness training	psychoeducation on the role of social competence in coping with binge eating, promoting children's coping with teasing
Weight management phase		
Balanced nutrition reduction of intake of fatty foods	dietary restriction, e.g. Traffic Light Diet [107, 108]	parents as providers of a balanced fat-reduced nutrition, family eating rules (e.g. parents provide balanced nutrition, children may eat as much or as little as they decide to)

Physical activity training	limitation of sedentary lifestyle, promoting lifestyle activity and exercise	limitation of sedentary behavior (e.g. daily TV watching, PC games, reading); promoting lifestyle activity (e.g. cycling, walking instead of taking the bus) and exercise (e.g. football, swimming, skating)	parents' training as role models for active behavior in every day live (e.g. analysis of obstacles, reinforcement plans for children's efforts in increasing physical activity and decreasing sedentary behavior) motivating children to engage regularly in sports
Maintenance phase			
Relapse prevention training	identification of and coping with risk situations	anticipation of future risk situations for binge eating and weight gain planning of future coping strategies	'normalizing' relapses as logical step in behavior change, anticipation of relapse situations, supervising children's coping techniques

studies suggest a genetic transmission of binge eating [13, 55–57]. For further details about research on genetic or psychosocial risk factors in the etiology of BED see also the chapter by Hilbert [this vol., pp. 149–164]. Future research may specify and replicate risk factors of BED [58], preferably using larger sample sizes and differentiating risk factors and early eating disorder symptoms.

Psychological Psychotherapy

Evidence on treatments for BED in childhood and adolescence is sparse. Clearly, the full spectrum of medical, nutritional, psychological, and social problems associated with BED symptomatology in children and adolescents represent indications for treatment and may need to be addressed by a multidisciplinary team. The development of treatment protocols may be guided by the growing body of evidence in the treatment of adults with BED, with cognitive-behavioral therapy being the most empirically supported treatment [59]. Concerning behavioral weight loss programs for childhood obesity, it remains unclear if these approaches are also successful in reducing symptoms of disordered eating [60].

Considering principles of the treatment of AN and BN in children, childhood obesity and BED in adults [61–67], the following guidelines for the treatment of BED in childhood refer to the treatment rationale 'treatment of the disordered eating before weight regulation' what seems to be the precondition for a stable weight reduction in adults [68, 69]. Therefore, in the initial phase of the treatment, children should learn to identify and change the triggering and maintaining cues of binge eating. For this purpose, they are taught to analyze target behavior by applying behavioral techniques such as self-monitoring, stimulus control and response prevention. Parents are trained in their role to support, promote, and supervise children's efforts, e.g. by providing a balanced and regular nutrition and reinforcement for behavior change. Behavioral weight management techniques and the parent's training have been shown to be effective in the treatment of childhood obesity [70–73]. Negative feelings as a result of interpersonal stressors are often mentioned as triggers for binge eating in adults [8]. Therefore, children are trained in social competence, especially self-assertiveness, and coping techniques [74].

For weight management purposes, the children in the second treatment phase, are advised to follow a balanced nutritional style and are reinforced (encouraged) to engage in regular physical activity. In the maintenance children and their parents are taught to identify lapses and prelapses in an early stage and to accept them as a natural step in behavior change [75]. For an example of a treatment protocol for BED in childhood, see table 5. In case of extreme obesity, hospitalization in a specialized clinical institution may be necessary [76; Braet, this vol., pp. 117–137]. Effectiveness of treatment of BED in childhood and adolescence according to these therapeutic guidelines remains to be evaluated in controlled clinical trials.

Implications for Future Research

About 1–3% of children and adolescents suffer from BED and the associated physical and psychological sequelae. The study of BED in childhood remains problematic for several reasons: The diagnostic validity of BED criteria has not yet been established in children and adolescents. Further, there is a lack of suitable assessment methods that are comparable across languages. Future epidemiological studies may address the course of childhood BED considering possible fluctuations in presentation. Also, controlled clinical trials on the treatment of BED in children and adolescents are still outstanding.

Considering the increasing prevalence of childhood obesity [77, 78], which appears to be associated with BED in adults [79], rising prevalence rates of childhood BED can be assumed. Successful treatment of BED in children and adolescents may stabilize weight or at least prevent further weight gain, as suggested by evidence on the treatment of adult BED [69].

References

1   American Psychiatric Association (APA): Diagnostic and Statistical Manual of Mental Disorders: DSM-IV. Washington, American Psychiatric Association, 1994.
2   Wilfley DE, Wilson GT, Agras WS: The clinical significance of binge eating disorder. Int J Eat Disord 2003;34(suppl):96–106.
3   Marcus MD, Kalarchian MA: Binge eating in children and adolescents. Int J Eat Disord 2003; 34(suppl):47–57.
4   Hilbert A, Munsch S: 'Binge-Eating'-Störung bei Kindern und Jugendlichen. Kindheit und Entwicklung. In revision.
5   Guss JL, Kissileff HR, Devlin MJ, Zimmerli E, Walsh BT: Binge size increases with body mass index in women with binge-eating disorder. Obes Res 2002;10:1021–1029.
6   Hsu LK, Mulliken B, McDonagh B, Krupa Das S, Rand W, Fairburn CG, Rolls B, McCrory MA, Saltzman E, Shikora S, Dwyer J, Roberts S: Binge eating disorder in extreme obesity. Int J Obes Relat Metab Disord 2002;26:1398–1403.
7   Raymond NC, Neumeyer B, Warren CS, Lee SS, Peterson CB: Energy intake patterns in obese women with binge eating disorder. Obes Res 2003;11:869–879.
8   Greeno CG, Wing RR, Shiffman S: Binge antecedents in obese women with and without binge eating disorder. J Consult Clin Psychol 2000;68:95–102.
9   Wolff GE, Crosby RD, Roberts JA, Wittrock DA: Differences in daily stress, mood, coping, and eating behavior in binge eating and nonbinge eating college women. Addict Behav 2000;25:205–216.
10 Binford RB, Pederson Mussell M, Peterson CB, Crow SJ, Mitchell JE: Relation of binge eating age of onset to functional aspects of binge eating in binge eating disorder. Int J Eat Disord 2004;35: 286–292.

11   Yanovski SZ: Binge eating disorder and obesity in 2003: Could treating an eating disorder have a positive effect on the obesity epidemic? Int J Eat Disord 2003;34(suppl):117–120.

12   Vamado PJ, Williamson DA, Bentz BG, Ryan DH, Rhodes SK, O'Neil PM, Sebastian SB, Barker SE: Prevalence of binge eating disorder in obese adults seeking weight loss treatment. Eat Weight Disord 1997;2:117–124.

13   Bulik CM, Sullivan PF, Kendler KS: Genetic and environmental contributions to obesity and binge eating. Int J Eat Disord 2003;33:293–298.

14   Morgan CM, Yanovski SZ, Nguyen TT, McDuffie J, Sebring NG, Jorge MR, Keil M, Yanovski JA: Loss of control over eating, adiposity, and psychopathology in overweight children. Int J Eat Disord 2002;31:430–441.

15   Niego SH, Pratt EM, Agras WS: Subjective or objective binge: Is the distinction valid? Int J Eat Disord 1997;22:291–298.

16   Pratt EM, Niego SH, Agras WS: Does the size of a binge matter? Int J Eat Disord 1998;24: 307–312.

17   Ackard DM, Neumark-Sztainer D, Story M, Perry C: Overeating among adolescents: Prevalence and associations with weight-related characteristics and psychological health. Pediatrics 2003;111: 67–74.

18   Tanofsky-Kraff M, Yanovski SZ, Wilfley DE, Marmarosh C, Morgan CM, Yanovski JA: Eating-disordered behaviors, body fat, and psychopathology in overweight and normal-weight children. J Consult Clin Psychol 2004;72:53–61.

19   Isnard P, Michel G, Frelut ML, Vila G, Falissard B, Naja W, Navarro J, Mouren-Simeoni MC: Binge eating and psychopathology in severely obese adolescents. Int J Eat Disord 2003;34: 235–243.

20   Decaluwe V, Braet C: Prevalence of binge-eating disorder in obese children and adolescents seeking weight-loss treatment. Int J Obes Relat Metab Disord 2003;27:404–409.

21   Luby JL, Heffelfinger AK, Mrakotsky C, Hessler MJ, Brown KM, Hildebrand T: Preschool major depressive disorder: Preliminary validation for developmentally modified DSM-IV criteria. J Am Acad Child Adolesc Psychiatry 2002;41:928–937.

22   Bryant-Waugh R, Lask B: Eating disorders in children. J Child Psychol Psychiatry 1995;36(2): 191–202.

23   Nicholls D, Chater R, Lask B: Children into DSM don't go: A comparison of classification systems for eating disorders in childhood and early adolescence. Int J Eat Disord 2000;28:317–324.

24   Whitaker A, Davies M, Shaffer D, Johnson J, Abrams S, Walsh BT, Kalikow K: The struggle to be thin: A survey of anorexic and bulimic symptoms in a non-referred adolescent population. Psychol Med 1989;19:143–163.

25   Childress AC, Brewerton TD, Hodges EL, Jarrell MP: The Kids' Eating Disorders Survey (KEDS): A study of middle school students. J Am Acad Child Adolesc Psychiatry 1993;32:843–850.

26   Field AE, Camargo CA Jr, Taylor CB, Berkey CS, Frazier AL, Gillman MW, Colditz GA: Overweight, weight concerns, and bulimic behaviors among girls and boys. J Am Acad Child Adolesc Psychiatry 1999;38:754–760.

27   Croll J, Neumark-Sztainer D, Story M, Ireland M: Prevalence and risk and protective factors related to disordered eating behaviors among adolescents: Relationship to gender and ethnicity. J Adolesc Health 2002;31:166–175.

28   Britz B, Siegfried W, Ziegler A, Lamertz C, Herpertz-Dahlmann BM, Remschmidt H, Wittchen HU, Hebebrand J: Rates of psychiatric disorders in a clinical study group of adolescents with extreme obesity and in obese adolescents ascertained via a population based study. Int J Obes Relat Metab Disord 2000;24:1707–1714.

29   Johnson WG, Rohan KJ, Kirk AA: Prevalence and correlates of binge eating in white and African American adolescents. Eat Behav 2002;3:179–189.

30   Decaluwe VV, Braet C: Assessment of eating disorder psychopathology in obese children and adolescents: Interview versus self-report questionnaire. Behav Res Ther 2004;42:799–811.

31   Bryant-Waugh RJ, Cooper PJ, Taylor CL, Lask BD: The use of the eating disorder examination with children: A pilot study. Int J Eat Disord 1996;19:391–397.

32   Stice E, Agras WS, Hammer LD: Risk factors for the emergence of childhood eating disturbances: A five-year prospective study. Int J Eat Disord 1999;25:375–387.

33   Steinhausen HC, Boyadjieva S, Griogoroiu-Serbanescu M, Neumarker KJ: The outcome of adolescent eating disorders: Findings from an international collaborative study. Eur Child Adolesc Psychiatry 2003;12(suppl 1):191–198.

34   Steinhausen HC, Rauss-Mason C, Seidel R: Follow-up studies of anorexia nervosa: A review of four decades of outcome research. Psychol Med 1991;21:447–454.

35   Kotler LA, Cohen P, Davies M, Pine DS, Walsh BT: Longitudinal relationships between childhood, adolescent, and adult eating disorders. J Am Acad Child Adolesc Psychiatry 2001;40:1434–1440.

36   Döpfner M, Lehmkuhl G, Heubrock D, Petermann F: Diagnostik psychischer Störungen im Kindes- und Jugendalter. Göttingen, Hogrefe, 2000.

37   Christie D, Watkins B, Lask B: Assessment; in Lask B, Bryant-Waugh R (eds): Anorexia nervosa and Related Eating Disorders in Childhood and Adolescence. Hove, Psychology Press Taylor & Francis, 2000, pp 105–125.

38   Neumark-Sztainer D, Story M: Dieting and binge eating among adolescents: What do they really mean? J Am Diet Assoc 1998;98:446–450.

39   Wilson GT: Assessment of binge eating; in Fairburn CG, Wilson GT (eds): Binge Eating: Nature, Assessment, and Treatment. New York, Guilford Press, 1993, pp 227–249.

40   Wilson GT, Vitousec KM: Self-Monitoring in the assessment of eating disorders. Psychol Assessment 1999;11:480–489.

41   Archer LA, Rosenbaum PL, Streiner DL: The children's eating behavior inventory: Reliability and validity results. J Pediatr Psychol 1991;16:629–642.

42   Johnson WG, Grieve FG, Adams CD, Sandy J: Measuring binge eating in adolescents: Adolescent and parent versions of the questionnaire of eating and weight patterns. Int J Eat Disord 1999;26: 301–314.

43   Fairburn CG, Doll HA, Welch SL, Hay PJ, Davies BA, O'Connor ME: Risk factors for binge eating disorder: A community-based, case-control study. Arch Gen Psychiatry 1998;55:425–432.

44   Spurrell EB, Wilfley DE, Tanofsky MB, Brownell KD: Age of onset for binge eating: Are there different pathways to binge eating? Int J Eat Disord 1997;21:55–65.

45   Abbott DW, de Zwaan M, Mussell MP, Raymond NC, Seim HC, Crow SJ, Crosby RD, Mitchell JE: Onset of binge eating and dieting in overweight women: Implications for etiology, associated features and treatment. J Psychosom Res 1998;44(3–4):367–374.

46   Grilo CM, Masheb RM: Onset of dieting vs binge eating in outpatients with binge eating disorder. Int J Obes Relat Metab Disord 2000;24:404–409.

47   Jackson TD, Grilo CM, Masheb RM: Teasing history, onset of obesity, current eating disorder psychopathology, body dissatisfaction, and psychological functioning in binge eating disorder. Obes Res 2000;8:451–458.

48   Neumark-Sztainer D, Falkner N, Story M, Perry C, Hannan PJ, Mulert S: Weight-teasing among adolescents: Correlations with weight status and disordered eating behaviors. Int J Obes Relat Metab Disord 2002;26:123–131.

49   Wardle J, Sanderson S, Guthrie CA, Rapoport L, Plomin R: Parental feeding style and the intergenerational transmission of obesity risk. Obes Res 2002;10:453–462.

50   Zaider TI, Johnson JG, Cockell SJ: Psychiatric comorbidity associated with eating disorder symptomatology among adolescents in the community. Int J Eat Disord 2000;28:58–67.

51   Birch LL, Fisher JO, Davison KK: Learning to overeat: Maternal use of restrictive feeding practices promotes girls' eating in the absence of hunger. Am J Clin Nutr 2003;78:215–220.

52   Laessle RG, Uhl H, Lindel B, Muller A: Parental influences on laboratory eating behavior in obese and non-obese children. Int J Obes Relat Metab Disord 2001;25(suppl 1):60–62.

53   Drucker RR, Hammer LD, Agras WS, Bryson S: Can mothers influence their child's eating behavior? J Dev Behav Pediatr 1999;20:88–92.

54   Klesges RC, Stein RJ, Eck LH, Isbell TR, Klesges LM: Parental influence on food selection in young children and its relationships to childhood obesity. Am J Clin Nutr 1991;53:859–864.

55   Fowler SJ, Bulik CM: Family environment and psychiatric history in women with binge-eating disorder and obese controls. Behav Change 1997;14:106–112.

56   Lee YH, Abbott DW, Seim H, Crosby RD, Monson N, Burgard M, Mitchell JE: Eating disorders and psychiatric disorders in the first-degree relatives of obese probands with binge eating disorder and obese non-binge eating disorder controls. Int J Eat Disord 1999;26:322–332.

57 Branson R, Potoczna N, Kral JG, Lentes KU, Hoehe MR, Horber FF: Binge eating as a major phenotype of melanocortin 4 receptor gene mutations. N Engl J Med 2003;348:1096–1103.

58 Jacobi C, Hayward C, de Zwaan M, Kraemer HC, Agras WS: Coming to terms with risk factors for eating disorders: Application of risk terminology and suggestions for a general taxonomy. Psychol Bull 2004;130:19–65.

59 Wilson GT, Fairburn CG: Eating disorders; in Nathan PE, Gorman JM (eds): A Guide to Treatments that Work. New York, Oxford University Press, 2002, pp 559–592.

60 Epstein LH, Paluch RA, Saelens BE, Ernst MM, Wilfley DE: Changes in eating disorder symptoms with pediatric obesity treatment. J Pediatr 2001;139:58–65.

61 Robin AL, Gilroy M, Dennis AB: Treatment of eating disorders in children and adolescents. Clin Psychol Rev 1998;18:421–446.

62 Powers PS, Santana CA: Childhood and adolescent anorexia nervosa. Child Adolesc Psychiatr Clin N Am 2002;11:219–235.

63 Brewerton TD: Bulimia in children and adolescents. Child Adolesc Psychiatr Clins N Am 2002; 11(viii):237–256.

64 Fairburn CG, Harrison PJ: Eating disorders. Lancet 2003;361:407–416.

65 Epstein LH, Myers MD, Raynor HA, Saelens BE: Treatment of pediatric obesity. Pediatrics 1998; 101:554–570.

66 Goldfield GS, Epstein LH: Management of obesity in children; in Fairburn CG, Brownell KD (eds): Eating Disorders and Obesity: A Comprehensive Handbook. New York, Guilford Press, 2002, pp 573–577.

67 Wonderlich SA, de Zwaan M, Mitchell JE, Peterson C, Crow S: Psychological and dietary treatments of binge eating disorder: Conceptual implications. Int J Eat Disord 2003;34(suppl):S58–S73.

68 Wilson GT: Cognitive behavior therapy for eating disorders: Progress and problems. Behav Res Ther 1999;37(suppl 1):79–95.

69 Wilfley DE, Welch RR, Stein RI, Spurrell EB, Cohen LR, Saelens BE, Dounchis JZ, Frank MA, Wiseman CV, Matt GE: A randomized comparison of group cognitive-behavioral therapy and group interpersonal psychotherapy for the treatment of overweight individuals with binge-eating disorder. Arch Gen Psychiatry 2002;59:713–721.

70 Epstein LH, Valoski A, Wing RR, McCurley J: Ten-year outcomes of behavioral family-based treatment for childhood obesity. Health Psychol 1994;13:373–383.

71 Petermann F, Grunewald L, Gartmann-Skambracks A, Warschburger P: Verhaltenstherapeutische Behandlung der kindlichen Adipositas. Kindh Entwickl 1999;8:206–217.

72 Warschburger P, Fromme C, Petermann F, Wojtalla N, Oepen J: Conceptualisation and evaluation of a cognitive-behavioural training programme for children and adolescents with obesity. Int J Obes Relat Metab Disord 2001;25(suppl 1):93–95.

73 McLean N, Griffin S, Toney K, Hardeman W: Family involvement in weight control, weight maintenance and weight-loss interventions: A systematic review of randomised trials. Int J Obes Relat Metab Disord 2003;27:987–1005.

74 Petermann F: Klinische Kinderpsychologie: Das Konzept der sozialen Kompetenz. Clinical child psychology: The concept of social competence. Z Psychol 2002;210:175–185.

75 Brownell KD: The LEARN Program for Weight Control. USA, American Health Publishing Company, 1997.

76 Braet C, Tanghe A, Bode PD, Franckx H, Winckel MV: Inpatient treatment of obese children: A multicomponent programme without stringent calorie restriction. Eur J Pediatr 2003;162:391–396.

77 Herpertz-Dahlmann B, Geller F, Bohle C, Khalil C, Trost-Brinkhues G, Ziegler A, Hebebrand J: Secular trends in body mass index measurements in preschool children from the City of Aachen, Germany. Eur J Pediatr 2003;162:104–109.

78 Ogden CL, Flegal KM, Carroll MD, Johnson CL: Prevalence and trends in overweight among US children and adolescents, 1999–2000. JAMA 2002;288:1728–1732.

79 Spitzer RL, Yanovski S, Wadden T, Wing R, Marcus MD, Stunkard A, Devlin M, Mitchell J, Hasin D, Horne RL: Binge eating disorder: Its further validation in a multisite study. Int J Eat Disord 1993; 13:137–153.

80 Ledoux S, Choquet M, Manfredi R: Associated factors for self-reported binge eating among male and female adolescents. J Adolesc 1993;16:75–91.

81   Kandel DB, Davies M: Epidemiology of depressive mood in adolescents: An empirical study. Arch Gen Psychiatry 1982;39:1205–1212.
82   Devaud C, Jeannin A, Narring F, Ferron C, Michaud PA: Eating disorders among female adolescents in Switzerland: Prevalence and associations with mental and behavioral disorders. Int J Eat Disord 1998;24:207–216.
83   Choquet M, Ledoux S: Les troubles des conduites alimentaires. Paris, INSERM, 1991.
84   Michaud P-A, Narring F: Methodological issues in adolescent health surveys: The case of the Swiss multicenter adolescent survey on health. Soz Präventivmed 1995;40:172–182.
85   Shisslak CM, Renger R, Sharpe T, Crago M, McKnight KM, Gray N, Bryson S, Estes LS, Parnaby OG, Killen J, Taylor CB: Development and evaluation of the McKnight Risk Factor Survey for assessing potential risk and protective factors for disordered eating in preadolescent and adolescent girls. Int J Eat Disord 1999;25:195–214.
86   Kann L, Warren CW, Harris WA, Collins JL, Williams BI, Ross JG, Kolbe LJ: Youth risk behavior surveillance – United States, 1995. J Sch Health 1996;66:365–377.
87   Saunders SM, Resnick MD, Hoberman HM, Blum RW: Formal help-seeking behavior of adolescents identifying themselves as having mental health problems. J Am Acad Child Adolesc Psychiatry 1994;33:718–728.
88   Johnston L, O'Malley P, Bachman J: The Monitoring the Future project after twenty two years: Design and procedures. Monitoring the Future Occasional Paper. Ann Arbor, Institute for Social Research, 1996.
89   Spitzer RL, Yanovski SZ, Marcus MD: Questionnaire on eating and weight patterns revised [QEWP R]; in Allison DB (ed): Handbook of Assessment Methods for Eating Behaviors and Weight-Related Problems: Measures, Theory, and Research. Thousand Oaks, Sage, 1995.
90   Berkowitz R, Stunkard AJ, Stallings VA: Binge-eating disorder in obese adolescent girls. Ann NY Acad Sci 1993;699:200–206.
91   Severi F, Verri A, Livieri C: Eating behaviour and psychological profile in childhood obesity. Adv Biosci 1993;90:329–336.
92   Wilson GT, Walsh BT: Eating disorders in the DSM-IV. J Abnorm Psychol 1991;100:362–365.
93   Wittchen H, Beloch E, Garczynski E, Holly A, Lachner G, Perkonigg A, Pfütze EM, Schuster P, Vodermaier A, Vossen A, Wunderlich U, Zieglgänsberger S: Münchener Composite International Diagnostic Interview (M-CIDI, Paper-pencil and CAPI version 2.2, 2 = 95, English). Munich, Max-Planck-Institut für Psychiatrie, Klinisches Institut, 1995.
94   Gormally J, Black S, Daston S, Rardin D: The assessment of binge eating severity among obese persons. Addict Behav 1982;7:47–55.
95   Decaluwe V, Braet C, Fairburn CG: Binge eating in obese children and adolescents. Int J Eat Disord 2003;33:78–84.
96   Fairburn CG, Beglin SJ: Assessment of eating disorders: Interview or self-report questionnaire? Int J Eat Disord 1994;16:363–370.
97   Fairburn CG, Cooper PJ: The Eating Disorder Examination; in Fairburn CG, Wilson GT (eds): Binge Eating: Nature, Assessment, and Treatment. New York, Guilford Press, 1993, pp 317–360.
98   Hilbert A, Tuschen-Caffier B, Ohms M: Eating Disorder Examination: Deutschsprachige Version des strukturierten Essstörungsinterviews. Diagnostica 2004;50:98–106.
99   Veron-Guidry S, Williamson DA: Development of a body image assessment procedure for children and preadolescents. Int J Eat Disord 1996;20:287–293.
100 Franzen S, Florin I: Der Dutch Eating Behavior Questionnaire für Kinder (DEBQ-K) – Ein Fragebogen zur Erfassung gezügelten Essverhaltens. Kindh Entwickl 1997;6:116–122.
101 Van Strien T, Frijters JE, Bergers GP, Defares PB: The Dutch Eating Behavior Questionnaire (DEBQ) for assessment of restrained, emotional, and external eating behavior. Int J Eat Disord 1986;5:195–315.
102 Carter JC, Stewart DA, Fairburn CG: Eating disorder examination questionnaire: Norms for young adolescent girls. Behav Res Ther 2001;39:625–632.
103 Masheb RM, Grilo CM: On the relation of attempting to lose weight, restraint, and binge eating in outpatients with binge eating disorder. Obes Res 2000;8:638–645.
104 Stice E, Presnell K, Spangler D: Risk factors for binge eating onset in adolescent girls: A 2-year prospective investigation. Health Psychol 2002;21:131–138.

Binge Eating Disorder in Childhood

105 Fisher JO, Birch LL: Restricting access to foods and children's eating. Appetite 1999;32:405–419.
106 Fisher JO, Birch LL: Restricting access to palatable foods affects children's behavioral response, food selection, and intake. Am J Clin Nutr 1999;69:1264–1272.
107 Epstein LH, Masek BJ, Marshall WR: A nutritionally based school program for control of eating in obese children. Behav Ther 1978;9:766–788.
108 Epstein LH, Paluch RA, Gordy CC, Saelens BE, Ernst MM: Problem solving in the treatment of childhood obesity. J Consult Clin Psychol 2000;68:717–721.

Dr. Simone Munsch
Institut für Klinische Psychologie und Psychotherapie
Universität Basel, Missionsstrasse 62a, CH–4055 Basel (Schweiz)
Tel. +41 61 267 06 57, Fax +41 61 267 06 48, E-Mail simone.munsch@unibas.ch

Munsch S, Beglinger C (eds): Obesity and Binge Eating Disorder.
Bibl Psychiatr. Basel, Karger, 2005, No 171, pp 197–216

....

Binge Eating Disorder: Specific and Common Features

A Comprehensive Overview

Simone Munsch, Kathrin Dubi

Institut für Psychologie, Universität Basel, Basel, Schweiz

While clinical features of the two officially recognized eating disorders anorexia nervosa (AN) and bulimia nervosa (BN) are well defined, questions still remain about the diagnostic features and the specific and associated psychopathology of BED in comparison to BN and obesity. Since the multisite field trials [1] empirical studies have reported general, but not unequivocal support for the validity of the BED diagnosis [2, 3]. Overall, people with BED differ from those who do not binge eat, and BED appears to have important similarities with and differences from BN [3]. The goal of this chapter is to provide a comprehensive overview of the profile of the clinical features associated with BED compared to BN and obesity. Understanding the similarities and differences among BN, BED and obesity might shed light onto the debate, whether or not BED forms a new diagnostic category, will facilitate diagnosis in clinical practice and might help tailor treatment strategies to individual cases.

We included studies published between 1990 and 2004 if they were empirically reviewed and included the comparison of at least two of the following groups, BED, BN and obesity (table 1). Subjects had to meet BED criteria according to DSM IV. Surveys of subclinical or subthreshold patients were excluded. Further we only included investigations about dietary and psychotherapeutic interventions and did not consider psychopharmacological therapies.

BED is often associated with overweight and obesity, as evidenced by findings from clinic, community, and population-based studies [1, 4, 45–49]. Measured or self-reported BMI of BED patients was higher than in BN patients in community-based studies [4, 17] and in the clinical population [5]. Self-reported and measured BMI of BED patients were similar to obese patients in

Table 1. Clinical characteristics of BED in comparison to BN and/or obesity

Methods	Authors	Sample and study characteristics N, a, BMI (kg/m²), Sex (f/m), long/CS, clin/comm
BMI		
BED > BN		
Measured	Fairburn et al. [4]	48 BED, a = 24.7, BMI = 25.5, 102 BN, a = 23.9, BMI = 24.4, f, clin, long
	Fitzgibbon and Blackman [5]	35 BED, a = 40.3, BMI = 41.1, 42 BN, a = 28.0, BMI = 23.5, f/m, clin, CS
Self-reported		
BED = Ob		
Measured	Gladis et al. [6]	14 BED, a = 42.1, BMI = 38.9, 59 Ob, a = 42.3, BMI = 36.3 f, clin, long
	Telch and Stice [7]	61 ob BED, a = 43.5, BMI = 34.8, 60 Ob, a = 45.0, BMI = 32.5, f, comm, CS
	Nauta et al. [8]	37 BED, 37 Ob, a = 38.3, BMI = 33.1, f, clin, long
Self-reported	Jirik-Babb and Geliebter [9]	21 BED, a = 43.5, BMI = 30.95, 22 Ob, a = 43.5, BMI = 34.64, f, clin, CS
	Eldredge and Agras [10]	35 ob BED, a = 39.7, BMI = 31.03, 53 ob EDNOS, a = 42.6, BMI = 32.34, 68 Ob, a = 39.0, BMI = 29.22, f, clin, CS
Eating behavior		
Restraint eating		
BED < BN		
EDE	Fairburn et al. [4]	
TFEQ	Brody et al. [11]	13 ob BED, a = 44.2, 55 BN, a = 25.4, 54 Ob, a = 42.7, f/m, clin, CS

Measure	Comparison	Reference	Sample
Res. Sc., TFEQ	BED = BN	Cooke et al. [12]	10 ob BED, a = 37.0, 10 Ob, a = 42.0, f, comm, CS
		Wilfley et al. [13]	105 ob BED, a = 45.5, 15 Ob, a = 27.2, 53 BN, a = 22.1, f, clin, CS
EDE-Q	BED = Ob	Masheb and Grilo [14]	51 ob BED, a = 43.6, non-ob BED, a = 37.3, 46 BN, a = 31.8, f, clin, CS
EDE-Q, QEWP-R TFEQ EDE	BED > Ob	Nauta et al. [8] Brody et al. [11] Wilfley et al. [13]	
Res. Sc., TFEQ		Goldfein et al. [15]	10 ob BED, a = 37.0, 10 Ob, a = 42.0, f, comm, CS
EDE-Q	Disinhibition BED = BN	Telch and Stice [7]	
TFEQ		Brody et al. [11]	
TFEQ	BED > Ob	Fichter et al. [16] Goldfein et al. [15]. Telch and Stice [7], Brody et al. [11]. Cooke et al. [12]	
EDE	Body concept Weight and shape concern BED > Ob	Eldredge and Agras [10], Wilfley et al. [13]	22 BED, a = 34.3, 22 BN, a = 33.3, 16 Ob, a = 33.5, f/m, clin, CS

Table 1 (continued)

Methods	Authors		Sample and study characteristics N, a, BMI (kg/m²), Sex (f/m), long/CS, clin/comm
EDE-Q	Telch and Stice [7], Nauta et al. [8], Masheb and Grilo [14]	Body dissatisfaction BED = BN	
EDI, EDE	Striegel-Moore et al. [17] Barry et al. [18]	BED > BN	79 ob BED, a = 42.7, 37 non-ob BED, a = 38.5, 46 PBN, a = 30.4, f, clin, CS
EDI	Fichter et al. [16]	BED = Ob	
EDI	Fassino et al. [19]	*Self-reported binges* Binge frequency BED = BN	51 ob BED (clin), a = 34.5, 52 Ob; (comm), a = 35.2, f, CS
EDE-Q	Masheb and Grilo [14]	Quantity and quality of binges BED = BN Binges of BED < BN (carbohydrates and sugar)	
QEWP-R, Food Processor for Windows Nutrition Analysis Software	Fitzgibbon and Blackman [5]		

Method	Reference	Findings	Sample
Telephone interviews/Nutrition Data System software	Raymond et al. [20]	BED > Ob (kcal)	12 ob BED, a = 37.9, 8 Ob, a = 34.9, f, clin, CS
Multicourse meals in laboratory	Yanovski et al. [21]	*Binges in laboratory setting* BED > Ob (kcal, binge/normal meal instructions) BED > Ob (fat intake) and < Ob (protein intake) Multi-item meal: BED > Ob (kcal) Single-item meal: BED = Ob	10 ob BED, a = 36.2, 9 Ob, a = 39.0, f, clin, CS
Instruction to binge	Goldfein et al. [15]	BED > Ob (meat intake) BED = Ob (food choices, time spent eating)	
Multiple-item meal, instruction to binge	Cooke et al. [12]	*Comorbidity* BED = BN (affective, anxiety disorders, substance abuse)	
SCID-IV	Striegel-Moore et al. [17]	BED > Ob (any lifetime axis I disorder,	

Table 1 (continued)

Methods	Authors	Sample and study characteristics N, a, BMI (kg/m²), Sex (f/m), long/CS, clin/comm
major depression, anxiety disorder, BN)		
SCID	Yanovski et al.[22]	43 ob BED, a = 36.1, 85 Ob, a = 37.2, f/m, clin, CS
SCID-IV	Telch and Stice [7] Fontenelle et al. [23]	33 ob BED, a = 34.1, 32 Ob, a = 36.1, f/m, clin, CS
(any lifetime axis II disorder, borderline, avoidant personality disorder)		
SCID-II	Yanovski et al. [22], Telch and Stice [7]	
BED = Ob (any lifetime axis I disorder, affective disorder, substance abuse/dependence)		
SCID	Brody et al. [11] Ricca et al. [24]	26 ob BED, 318 Ob, a = 43.5, f/m, clin, CS
General psychopathology Depressive feelings BED < BN		
BDI	Barry et al. [18], Brody et al. [11]	

Measure	Result	Studies	Sample
HAM-D BDI, SCL-90	BED = BN	Crow et al. [25] Tobin et al. [26]	122 BED, 142 BN, a = ?, f, clin, CS 31 BED, a = 31, 188 PBN, a = 25, 21 NBN, a = 32, f/m, clin, CS
BDI	BED > Ob	Yanovski et al. [27] Fichter et al. [16], Telch and Stice [7], Gladis et al. [6], Nauta et al. [8], Fassino et al. [19], Jirik-Babb and Geliebter [9], Fontenelle et al. [23]	21 ob BED, a = 36, 17 Ob, a = 36, f, clin, long
BDI	BED = Ob	Ricca et al. [24], Brody et al. [11]	
SCL-90	*Anxiety* BED < BN	Tobin et al. [26]	
BAI STAI	BED = Ob	Jirik-Babb and Geliebter [9] Ricca et al. [24]	
SELF-reported, retrospective	*Age of onset of overweight/obesity* BED = BN	Fichter et al. [16]	
BDI	BED = Ob	Fichter et al. [16], Yanovski et al. [21], Goldfein et al. [15], Telch and Stiche [7], Eldredge	

Table 1 (continued)

Methods	Authors	Sample and study characteristics N, a, BMI (kg/m²), Sex (f/m), long/CS, clin/comm
BED < Ob (age of onset)	and Agras [10], Nauta et al. [8], Fassino et al. [19]	
	Johnsen et al. [28] Brody et al. [11], Yanovski et al. [27]	199 ob BED, 65 Ob, A = 44.7, f, clin, CS
Age of onset of eating disorder BED = BN	Fairburn et al. [4]	
Self-reported, retrospective		
Treatment effectiveness Weight loss during treatment BED > Ob	Gladis et al. [6]	
BED = Ob	Raymond et al. [29]	63 ob BED, a = 39.3, 29 Ob, a = 38.8, f, clin, long
	Yanovski et al. [27], Nauta et al. [8], Jirik-Babb and Geliebter [9]	
Weight regain BED = Ob	Gladis et al. [6], Raymond et al. [29] Nauta et al. [8]	
BED > Ob Depressiveness, eating behavior, body dissatisfaction BED > Ob, restraint: BED = Ob		
BDI, EDE-Q, QEWP-R	Nauta et al. [8]	

	Natural course binge frequency	
5-year fu: BN > BED Brief Sym. Inv., SCID		Fairburn et al. [4]
5-year fu: BED > BN Brief Sym. Inv., SCID	remission	Fairburn et al. [4]
5-year fu: BED < BN (major depression, anxiety disorder) Brief Sym. Inv., SCID	Comorbidity	Fairburn et al. [4]
5-year fu: BED < BN (alcohol abuse), BED > BN (self esteem) Brief Sym. Inv., SEQ	Psychopathological symptoms	Fairburn et al. [4]
5-year fu: ↓ of weight, shape, eating concern, restraint: BED = BN EDE	Disturbed eating behavior/ body dissatisfaction	Fairburn et al. [4]

a = Age; BAI = Beck Anxiety Inventory [30]; BDI = Beck Depression Inventory [31]; BED = binge eating disorder; BMI = Body Mass Index; BN = bulimia nervosa; Brief Sym. Inv. = Brief Symptom Inventory [32]; clin = clinical population (treatment seeking individuals); comm = community sample; CS = cross-sectional study; EDE = eating disorder examination [33]; EDE-Q = Eating Disorder Examination – Questionnaire [34]; EDI = Eating Disorder Inventory [35]; f = female; fu = follow-up; HAM-D = Hamilton Depression Scale [36]; long = longitudinal study; m = male; N = sample size; Ob = obesity; Res. Sc. = Restraint Scale [37]; QEWP-R = Questionnaire of Eating and Weight Patterns – Revised [1]; SCID = Structured Clinical Interview for DSM-III-R [38]; SCID-II = Structured Clinical Interview for DSM-III-R Personality Disorders [39]; SCID-IV = Structured Clinical Interview for DSM-IV Axis I Disorders [40]; SCL-90 = Hopkins Symptom Checklist [41]; SEQ = Robson Self-Esteem Questionnaire [42]; STAI = State-Trait-Anxiety Inventory [43]; TFEQ = Three-Factor Eating Questionnaire [44]; < = significantly lower; > = significantly higher; ↓ = significant reduction; = = no significant differences.

clinical and community-based populations (ranging from 20.4 to 45.2) [6, 9, 10, 50]. Other workgroups confirm these results (e.g. [16, 18] for the comparison of BED and BN or Fassino et al. [19] for the comparison of BED and obesity). Data on the differences in BMI in BN and BED are limited by methodological problems. Several studies in fact report BMI but do not specify whether BMI was assessed by self-report or if it was directly measured [14, 16, 18, 19]. Furthermore, little is known about the accuracy of measured vs. self-reported BMI among overweight subjects although there seems to be some evidence that self-reported and measured BMI highly correlate [51]. Studies which investigate the difference between BED, BN and obesity in clinical and community-based samples which compare self-reported and measured BMIs and account for the influence of several other factors which might influence patients current BMI (age, sex and age of onset of the disorder) could clarify open questions.

If we compare the clinical features of eating behavior of BED, BN, and obese patients there are different results, depending on the instruments and the populations with and in which restraint or disinhibited eating are measured. Reviews of eating disorder assessment instruments conclude that the EDE is the method of choice when assessing the specific psychopathology of eating disorders [52]. Restraint eating (measured by EDE or EDE-Q) is expressed to a higher extent by patients with BN than with BED in clinical populations [4, 11, 13, 14]. The EDE-Q assesses both intent to restrict calories and actual efforts to restrain food intake. In a small community-based sample, where restraint eating was measured with the Herman and Mack's RS, no difference between BN and BED patients revealed [12]. Further, in clinical populations BED patients seem to exhibit a similar tendency as obese patients to restrain their eating behavior measured by EDE, EDE-Q and QEWP-R [8, 11, 13]. Others [7, 15] compared BED with obese patients in the community and showed a higher expressed restraint eating in the BED than in the obesity group measured with the RS, TFEQ and EDE-Q. Wilfley et al. [13] conclude that BED patients, compared to BN and AN individuals, exhibit a significantly lower score on the Restraint subscales. Extreme dietary restraint (e.g. going for a whole day without eating any food at all for having a completely empty stomach) seems to be a part of the characteristic psychopathology for AN and BN patients, but not for BED patients. Several findings indicate that the diet related behaviors and attitudes which form the restraint eating behavior are associated with obesity rather than with BED [13, 53].

Patients with BED in clinical and community samples exhibit a more expressed tendency to disinhibit their eating than obese subjects as it is shown by Fichter et al. [16], Goldfein et al. [15], Cooke et al. [12], Telch and Stice [7] and Brody et al. [11]. Feelings of hunger, the fear of loss of control [13] and disinhibition [54, 55] are markedly expressed in patients with BED and it can be hypothesized that these represent a special eating style of BED patients [20, 56–59].

In contrast to AN and BN, the research criteria for BED do not include cognitive distortions such as the overimportance of shape and weight in self-evaluation. The reason for this exclusion is unclear and it can be speculated that this omission may relate to uncertainty regarding the influence of weight status on weight and shape overconcern [10]. However, self-report and interview-based data of many work groups [7, 8, 10, 13, 14, 53] suggest that BED patients in clinical and community samples, as compared to non-BED obese patients, are much more concerned about their body weight and shape and that their self-esteem is regulated in the extreme by these aspects of their appearance. Wilfley et al. [13] show that BED and BN score highest on Weight and Shape Concern subscales of EDE, followed by significantly lower scores for AN patients, over-weight controls and normal-weight controls. Altogether this suggests that an additional diagnostic criterion reflecting the overimportance of weight and shape in self-evaluation may be as relevant for BED as it is for AN and BN [17]. Results regarding body dissatisfaction assessed with the EDI are less clear [16, 18, 19].

In a review on several self-report questionnaire measures to assess binge eating and associated symptomatology [53] several limitations emerged. For example, the terms 'binge' and 'binge eating' are not defined for the individual completing the questionnaire, most measures do not clear-cutly measure binge eating and they do not specify a consistent time frame for the occurrence of binge eating. The EDE-Q addresses these shortcomings and yields significant correlations with the corresponding EDE scores (Dietary Restraint, Eating Concern, Weight and Shape Concern) but the EDE-Q subscales were significantly higher than the EDE scores [60]. To our knowledge, there are no studies comparing the validity of the subscales of the Eating Disorder Inventory (EDI) with the subscales of EDE or EDE-Q. Therefore, it is unclear if the EDI sub-scale Body Dissatisfaction measures the same features as EDE subscale Shape Concern. The different expressions of body dissatisfaction might also reflect a greater variability of BED patients, which is mentioned in literature [61]. However, the need for weight concern as a additional clinical feature and diag-nostic criteria of BED is further supported by findings demonstrating that weight dissatisfaction in BED decreases as frequency of binge eating decreases, even when BMI does not change [62].

Recurrent episodes of binge eating are the salient behavioral characteristic of BED and BN. The frequency of self-reported binges in BN and BED seems to be comparable (ca. 17 in BED and 16 in BN binge eating episodes during 28 days) [14].

In practice, most clinical assessments of the amount of food consumed rely on self-report. Using food diaries the self-reported quantity and quality of food during binge eating seem to differ between obese and BED patients. BED patients have a greater caloric intake than obese controls [20]. The authors also found significant differences in the timing of nutrient intake throughout the day between the BED groups on binge days (binge >1,000 kcal) and the obese control group. BED group ate significantly more in the evening on binge days than their obese control group. Further the results indicate that the BED group ate more of all three major nutrient groups (protein, carbohydrate, and fat) on binge days than on non-binge days. However, the proportion of dietary calories from each of the nutrients shifted on BED binge days compared with non-binge days to favor consumption of fat over carbohydrates [20]. In a recent self-report study on the quantity and quality of binge eating episodes in BED and BN subjects [5], no overall difference in the kilocalorie intake between the two groups was revealed. When the nutritional content of the binges was analyzed, a difference was found in carbohydrate intake, with the BN group consuming more carbohydrates and sugar than the BED group. There was no difference in the amount of protein or fat intake between the two groups. There is good reason for concern about the accuracy of self-reports of food consumption. While obese patients might underestimate caloric intake [63], BED patients might overestimate the amount of eaten food because of their low self-esteem and distress that routinely accompanies BED [64].

Under controlled laboratory conditions BED patients who are either instructed to binge or to eat normally in multicourse meals ingested more calories than obese patients [15, 21]. In the single item meal condition, there was no difference between obese and BED patients regarding the amount of eaten kilocalories or rate of eating or duration of meal [15]. When asked to let themselves go and binge eat, not only did the BED patients consume almost 950 kcal more than obese controls, but their meal macronutrient composition also differed, consisting of a greater percentage of fat and a lesser percentage of protein, with equal amounts of carbohydrate. Although BED subjects often describe carbohydrate craving during binges, it appears that highly palatable foods that are high in fat as well as high in carbohydrate or protein are more often chosen [21]. A more recent study [12] found no differences between obese and BED patients regarding food choices or time spent in a laboratory eating a multi-item meal with the instruction to binge eat. No single study has conducted a direct comparison between BN and BED regarding binge episodes. However, in several studies, identical methods were used to examine the eating behavior of BED and BN subjects. Several differences were revealed: BN patients had a greater amount of caloric intake than BED patients. Under normal meal instructions BN subjects consumed fewer calories than the BED group or controls and finally, BN patients exhibited a more disordered food consumption than BED patients [64]. However, several questions remain unanswered. A major issue is whether the differences measured in laboratory exist outside this controlled setting or whether the observed differences are more reflective of a difference in behavioral response to a laboratory setting than of a real existing difference in a variety of environments.

Studies comparing point and lifetime prevalence rates of comorbid mental disorders of individuals with BED and BN found that BED patients exhibit less comorbid psychopathology, report less subjective distress and better social adjustment than those with BN [65]. Especially for affective disorders, several authors found higher current and lifetime prevalence rates in patients with BN when compared with BED subjects [66]. In another population-based study, the examination of the frequency of nine specific current or lifetime psychiatric diagnoses found no significant differences between BN and BED groups regarding current affective, anxiety, substance use and obsessive compulsive disorders. Moreover the groups did not differ in the lifetime prevalence of having at least one Axis I disorder [17]. Furthermore, Telch and Stice [7] showed that BED individuals are three times more likely to suffer from current major depressive disorder than an overweight non-eating-disordered sample. Several studies [7, 22, 23] underline that in a clinical sample, BED is associated with a greater relative risk for lifetime comorbid mental disorders on Axis I or II. Two other studies [11, 24] observed no significant difference in the lifetime prevalence rate of Axis I mental disorders between obese patients and BED individuals. This might partly be due to different types of recruitments, assessments and to small sample sizes. Generally, it is important to consider that BED patients are not only obese subjects with a comorbid mental disorder. Thus, the increased comorbidity among BED subjects is accounted for by the severity of binge eating and not by the degree of obesity [67].

BN and BED are additionally associated with psychopathological symptoms such as depressive symptoms. Discriminant analysis demonstrates that on the vast majority of items, BED and BN do not differ significantly [26]. In HAM-D only gastrointestinal symptoms, paranoid symptoms and obsessional symptoms distinguish BED from BN subjects. Each of the three scales scores are higher in the BN than in the BED group [25]. A recent investigation underlines that BN is associated with greater psychological disturbance than BED. Overall, patients with BN show higher BDI depression scores [11, 18]. There are several limitations to these results, e.g. the ratings were made by different clinicians and the samples all stem from BED and BN subjects who sought treatment at specialized centers. It remains open whether the results are generalizable to people with these eating disorders not seeking treatment or who seek treatment in nonspecialty clinics [26]. Several studies indicate that BED subjects have significantly higher depression scores than obese subjects without eating disorders [6, 7, 16, 19]. Also in the study of Ricca et al. [24], where no differences in depressed mood (BDI) were found, the relevant association between binge eating and psychopathology was confirmed. BED patients seem to suffer less from anxiety symptoms in SCL-90 than BN patients [26] and cannot be differentiated from an obese patient group using the BAI or STAI [9, 24]. These results rely on self-report assessments in mostly female samples. For further studies it would be useful to include both clinician-rated and self-rated measures and also consider male samples. Further investigations on general psychopathology in BN, BED, and obesity show that in a community-based cohort [4] and in clinical samples [8, 9, 19] BED patients are less affected from feelings of low self-esteem than BN, but show lower self-esteem than obese subjects. BED subjects also exhibit higher levels of anger, an angrier temperament, and a greater tendency toward the external expression of anger than obese samples. The tendency to impulsively express anger toward the external environment and people, which is typical of borderline personalities, emerges as the strongest discriminating element between obese patients and BED patients [19].

Several clinical or community-based studies find no differences in age of onset of obesity between BED and obese patients. Age of onset of obesity in the BED and obese populations varies from about 8.4 to 14.5 years of age, respectively [16], between around 12.3 and 16.6 years [21] or older [7, 8, 10, 15, 19]. Others report an earlier onset of obesity in BED than in obese samples [11, 27, 28, 68]. Only one study compared the age of onset of BED and BN patient samples [16] and found no differences. There is a very important caveat that should be borne in mind when interpreting these findings. First of all, patients are recalling retrospective information regarding age of overweight or obesity. Only prospective studies will provide objective information about measured weight and height at the onset of obesity. Second, although some samples were based in the community [15, 28] the findings are limited to women in the community who respond to treatment studies of binge eating and/or weight loss, rather than to examine characteristics associated with binge eating among women in the community. Only few studies have examined the chronology of the onset of binge eating, dieting, BED, and obesity. Results indicate that in BED the onset of binge eating frequently begins in the absence of prior dietary restraint or weight loss [see chapter by Hilbert in this volume, pp. 149–164]. About half of the patients with BED first start binge eating in the absence of dieting [69]. The only study investigating the onset of eating disorder in BED and other patient groups [4] just find a tendency for those with BN to be younger at the onset of their eating disorder (15.7 vs. 17.2). Furthermore, BN individuals were more likely to have ever received treatment for an eating disorder (26 vs. 5%) than the BED cohort.

Several studies try to clarify the role of binge eating in treatment outcome in trials with dietary interventions and exercise and find that BED patients achieve similar [9, 29] or even a greater weight loss [6] during treatment than obese patients. BED subjects did not differ from the obese patient group in their average weight gain at 1-year follow-up [6, 29]. The referred above-mentioned studies underline that caloric restriction does not worsen BED symptoms. This fact is consistent with the findings that dieting is not the precipitant of binge eating in all BED individuals. BED diagnosis was further clearly associated with weight gain during the 1-year follow-up period after treatment. This result strengthens the finding that stopping binge eating behavior is essential to maintain weight loss and prevent weight gain in individuals with BED [70]. Psychotherapeutic approaches to BED treatment produce a binge eating abstinence rate of about 50% at the 12-month follow-up [for an overview, see ref. 71], but achieve minimal effects on weight loss at 12-month follow-up. The most consistent finding was that regardless of treatment approach long-term weight loss was predicted by long-term binge eating status. Dietary approaches to treatment which do not specially target binge eating result in similar abstinence rates at 12-month follow-up (e.g. 33% in de Zwaan et al. [66]; 56% in Raymond et al. [29]). However, definitions and measurements of abstinence vary substantially across studies. Longer-term follow-up studies are needed and to clarify the stability of the abstinence from binge eating outcome in different treatment types.

In a recent study [8], obese binge eaters improved more for Shape, Weight Eating concern and the variables depression and self-esteem than obese non-binge eaters during a cognitive therapy. Restraint eating as measured with the EDE-Q was similar after treatment for obese and BED patients. This result was also found in similar investigations in which the EDE-Restraint subscale was used [53]. After treatment the level of restraint was increased in the behavioral treatment, while binge eating was reduced. Further investigation of the complex relationship between binge eating, chaotic eating patterns, and restraint in binge eaters seems warranted [8].

A further outcome variable of the treatment of BED is the drop-out rate of BED and obese patients. Drop-out rates from psychotherapy studies and dietary approaches amount overall to around 20% and the presence of binge eating does not seem to confer a greater risk of drop-out compared to obese individuals [71].

The first prospective study to compare the long-term course and outcome of BED and BN [4] indicates that over a 5-year period the frequency of binge eating declined to a lesser extent in the BN cohort (56%) than in the binge eating disorder group (77%). The outcome of the BED group was better, with 18% having a clinical eating disorder of some form, compared with 51% in the BN cohort. There was an increase in weight and BMI in both cohorts with the BED group remaining heavier and showing a tendency for a greater proportion to have a BMI of 30 or higher. At follow-up 41% of the BN cohort met DSM-III-R criteria for major depression compared with 23% of the BED group. The rates of anxiety disorder diagnoses were similar at 15% in the BN and 11% in the BED group. Psychopathological symptoms such as self-esteem scores did not change significantly in the BN group, but improved in the BED cohort, resulting in a higher score in the BED group. There were no significant changes in social adjustment, with the BED group continuing to function at a better level [4]. Both cohorts reduced their level of dietary restraint with the result that the groups were no longer significantly different at follow-up. The levels of concern about shape, weight and eating also decreased to an equivalent extent in both groups. Overall, the binge eating group resembled clinical samples with the disorder except that they had a lower BMI, which may be due to the younger age of this community-based sample.

The main finding of this study is that BED and BN had a different course and outcome over 5 years of prospective follow-up, while there was little movement between the two diagnostic categories. The outcome of those with BED was favorable in comparison with the BN cohort. In one respect their outcome was worse: not only did they start at a higher weight but they remained heavier over the 5 years with 39% eventually meeting criteria for obesity (20% in the BN group). The explanation for this weight gain is unclear, especially since there was a marked decrease in the frequency of binge eating. The outcome of this study is comparable to a 6-month follow-up of a community-based sample in New England in which it was found that half of those reassessed no longer had a BED [62]. The fluctuation in the BN group was much higher than in the BED sample. Each year about a third of the BN individuals remitted and a further third relapsed. Instability was also observed in the only other detailed prospective study of the course of BN [72]. In contrast, there was little flux among the BED group, where about 50% of participants remitting each year and few relapsed. Interpreting these results one has to bear in mind that several processes besides natural course, such as regression to the mean, life events and treatment are likely to have influenced course and outcome of BN and BED individuals.

Considering the state of research about shared and different features of BED with other eating disorders and obesity, there is still much debate as to whether or not it is justified to give BED the status of a distinct diagnostic entity. It has been argued that adding this new diagnosis carries the risk of 'trivializing the whole construct of mental disorders' since approximately 30% of obese weight loss participants might receive such a diagnosis [73]. There are several cautions regarding the argument that BED is a trivial diagnosis (i.e. responding to minimal interventions, fluctuation course, high placebo rates). The placebo rate of BED is comparable to that of depression (30–50% [64]), also other illnesses show long periods of remission (e.g. asthma, rheumatism) and moreover other disorders with spontaneous remission such as hay fewer benefit from symptomatic and preventive treatment. Cooper and Fairburn [74] propose to revise diagnostic criteria to minimize confusion in the diagnostic process as follows: A 3-month frame should be used to adapt the BED criteria to those of other eating disorders such as AN and BN. To render the scheme for making eating disorder diagnoses more coherent, episodes of binge eating in BED should be 'clearly distinguishable' from other forms of overeating. Further they propose that binge eating should not occur in 'the context of more than three episodes of self-induced vomiting or laxative misuse or sustained and marked dietary restriction designed to control body shape or weight' [74] to distinguish BED from the purging form of BN. Today expert groups underline that the diagnosis of BED is significant and important for several reasons: Individuals with BED differ from individuals without eating disorders and share similarities but differ from individuals with AN or BN. BED is not just a subtype of obesity. BED is associated with co-occurring physical and mental illnesses, as well as impaired quality of life and social functioning and constitutes an eating disorder of clinical severity and a significant public health problem.

Finally and most importantly the phenomenon of uncompensated binge eating exists and troubles those who experience it. Whether or not the current categorization as BED is appropriate will be revealed by further research, leading to an empirically based understanding that will improve treatment and prevention strategies.

References

1   Spitzer RL, Yanovski S, Wadden T, Wing R, Marcus MD, Stunkard A, Devlin M, Mitchell J, Hasin D, Horne RL: Binge eating disorder: Its further validation in a multisite study. Int J Eat Disord 1993;13:137–153.
2   Grilo CM: The assessment and treatment of binge eating disorder. J Pract Psychiatry Behav Hlth 1998;4:191–201.
3   Grilo CM: Binge eating disorder; in Fairburn CG, Brownell K (eds): Eating Disorder and Obesity. New York, Guilford Press, 2002, pp 178–182.
4   Fairburn CG, Cooper Z, Doll HA, Norman P, O'Connor M: The natural course of bulimia nervosa and binge eating disorder in young women. Arch Gen Psychiatry 2000;57:659–665.
5   Fitzgibbon ML, Blackman LR: Binge eating disorder and bulimia nervosa: Differences in the quality and quantity of binge eating episodes. Int J Eat Disord 2000;27:238–243.
6   Gladis MM, Wadden TA, Vogt R, Foster G, Kuehnel RH, Bartlett SJ: Behavioral treatment of obese binge eaters: Do they need different care? J Psychosom Res 1998;44:375–334.
7   Telch CF, Stice E: Psychiatric comorbidity in women with binge eating disorder: Prevalence rates from a non-treatment-seeking sample. J Consult Clin Psychol 1998;66:768–776.
8   Nauta H, Hospers H, Kok G, Jansen A: A comparison between a cognitive and a behavioral treatment for obese binge eaters and obese non-binge eaters. Behav Ther 2000;31:441–461.

9   Jirik-Babb P, Geliebter A: Comparison of psychological characteristics of binging and nonbinging obese, adult, female outpatients. Eat Weight Disord 2003;8:173–177.

10   Eldredge KL, Agras WS: Weight and shape overconcern and emotional eating in binge eating disorder. Int J Eat Disord 1996;19:73–82.

11   Brody ML, Walsh BT, Devlin MJ: Binge eating disorder: Reliability and validity of a new diagnostic category. J Consult Clin Psychol 1994;62:381–386.

12   Cooke EA, Guss JL, Kissileff HR, Devlin MJ, Walsh BT: Patterns of food selection during binges in women with binge eating disorder. Int J Eat Disord 1997;22:187–193.

13   Wilfley DE, Schwartz MB, Spurrell EB, Fairburn CG: Using the eating disorder examination to identify the specific psychopathology of binge eating disorder. Int J Eat Disord 2000;27:259–269.

14   Masheb RM, Grilo CM: Binge eating disorder: A need for additional diagnostic criteria. Compr Psychiatry 2000;41:159–162.

15   Goldfein JA, Walsh BT, LaChaussee JL, Kissileff HR, Devlin MJ: Eating behavior in binge eating disorder. Int J Eat Disord 1993;14:427–431.

16   Fichter MM, Quadflieg N, Brandl B: Recurrent overeating: An empirical comparison of binge eating disorder, bulimia nervosa, and obesity. Int J Eat Disord 1993;14:1–16.

17   Striegel-Moore RH, Cachelin FM, Dohm FA, Pike KM, Wilfley DE, Fairburn CG: Comparison of binge eating disorder and bulimia nervosa in a community sample. Int J Eat Disord 2001;29:157–165.

18   Barry DT, Grilo CM, Masheb RM: Comparison of patients with bulimia nervosa, obese patients with binge eating disorder, and nonobese patients with binge eating disorder. J Nerv Ment Dis 2003; 191:589–594.

19   Fassino S, Leombruni P, Piero A, Abbate-Daga G, Giacomo Rovera G: Mood, eating attitudes, and anger in obese women with and without Binge Eating Disorder. J Psychosom Res 2003;54:559–566.

20   Raymond NC, Neumeyer B, Warren CS, Lee SS, Peterson CB: Energy intake patterns in obese women with binge eating disorder. Obes Res 2003;11:869–879.

21   Yanovski SZ, Leet M, Yanovski JA, Flood M, Gold PW, Kissileff HR, Walsh BT: Food selection and intake of obese women with binge-eating disorder. Am J Clin Nutr 1992;56:975–980.

22   Yanovski SZ, Nelson JE, Dubbert BK, Spitzer RL: Association of binge eating disorder and psychiatric comorbidity in obese subjects. Am J Psychiatry 1993;150:1472–1479.

23   Fontenelle LF, Vitor Mendlowicz M, de Menezes GB, Papelbaum M, Freitas SR, Godoy-Matos A, Coutinho W, Appolinario JC: Psychiatric comorbidity in a Brazilian sample of patients with binge-eating disorder. Psychiatry Res 2003;119:189–194.

24   Ricca V, Mannucci E, Moretti S, Di Bernardo M, Zucchi T, Cabras PL, Rotella CM: Screening for binge eating disorder in obese outpatients. Compr Psychiatry 2000;41:111–115.

25   Crow SJ, Zander KM, Crosby RD, Mitchell JE: Discriminant function analysis of depressive symptoms in binge eating disorder, bulimia nervosa, and major depression. Int J Eat Disord 1996;19:399–404.

26   Tobin DL, Griffing A, Griffing S: An examination of subtype criteria for bulimia nervosa. Int J Eat Disord 1997;22:179–186.

27   Yanovski SZ, Gormally JF, Leser MS, Gwirtsman HE, Yanovski JA: Binge eating disorder affects outcome of comprehensive very-low-calorie diet treatment. Obes Res 1994;2:205–212.

28   Johnsen LA, Gorin A, Stone AA, le Grange D: Characteristics of binge eating among women in the community seeking treatment for binge eating or weight loss. Eat Behav 2003;3:295–305.

29   Raymond NC, de Zwaan M, Mitchell JE, Ackard D, Thuras P: Effect of a very low calorie diet on the diagnostic category of individuals with binge eating disorder. Int J Eat Disord 2002;31:49–56.

30   Beck AT, Steer RA: Beck Anxiety Inventory Manual. Psychological Corporation. San Antonio, Harcourt Brace, 1993.

31   Beck AT, Steer RA: Beck Depression Inventory. Psychological Corporation. New York, Harcourt Brace Janovitch, 1987.

32   Derogatis LR, Spencer PM: Brief Symptom Inventory: Administration, Scoring, and Procedure Manual. Baltimore, Clinical Psychometric Research, 1982.

33   Fairburn CG, Cooper Z: The Eating Disorders Examination; in Fairburn CG, Wilson GT (eds): Binge Eating: Nature, Assessment and Treatment. New York, Guilford Press, 1993, pp 160–192.

34   Fairburn CG, Beglin SJ: Assessment of eating disorders: Interview or self-report questionnaire? Int J Eat Disord 1994;16:363–370.

35 Garner DM, Olmstead MP, Polivy J: Development and validation of a multidimensional eating disorder inventory for anorexia nervosa and bulimia. Int J Eat Disord 1983;2:15–34.

36 Hamilton M: A rating scale for depression. J Neurol Neurosurg Psychiatry 1960;23:56–62.

37 Herman CP, Mack D: Restrained and unrestrained eating. J Pers 1975;43:647–660.

38 Spitzer RL, Williams JBW, Gibbon M, First MB: Structured Clinical Interview for DSM-III-R, Patient Edition/Non-patient Edition (SCID-P/SCID-NP). Washington, American Psychiatric Press, 1990.

39 Spitzer RL, Williams JBW, Gibbon M, First MB: Structured Clinician Interview for DSM-III-R Axis II Disorders (SCID-II). Washington, American Psychiatric Press, 1990.

40 First MB, Spitzer RL, Gibbon M, Williams JBW: Structured Clinical Interview for DSM-IV Axis I disorders. New York, Biometrics Research Department, New York State Psychiatric Institute, 1995.

41 Derogatis LR, Rickels K, Rock AF: The SCL-90 and the MMPI: A step in the validation of a new self-report scale. Br J Psychiatry 1976;128:280–289.

42 Robson P: Development of a new self-report questionnaire to measure self esteem. Psychol Med 1989;19:513–518.

43 Spielberger CD, Gorsuch RL, Lushene RE: Manual for the State-Trait Anxiety Inventory. Palo Alto, Consultant Psychologists Press, 1970.

44 Stunkard AJ, Messick S: The three-factor eating questionnaire to measure dietary restraint, disinhibition and hunger. J Psychosom Res 1985;29:71–83.

45 Bruce B, Agras WS: Binge eating in females: A population-based investigation. Int J Eat Disord 1992;12:365–373.

46 Smith DE, Marcus MD, Lewis CE, Fitzgibbon M, Schreiner P: Prevalence of binge eating disorder, obesity, and depression in a biracial cohort of young adults. Ann Behav Med 1998;20:227–232.

47 Spitzer RL, Devlin MJ, Walsh BT, Hasin D, Wing R, Marcus MD, Stunkard A, Wadden T, Yanovski S, Agras WS, Nonas C: Binge eating disorder: A multisite field trial of the diagnostic criteria. Int J Eat Disord 1992;11:191–203.

48 Striegel-Moore RH, Wilfley DE, Pike KM, Dohm FA, Fairburn CG: Recurrent binge eating in black American women. Arch Fam Med 2000;9:83–87.

49 Yanovski SZ: Binge eating in obese persons; in Fairburn CG, Brownell K (eds): Eating Disorders and Obesity, vol 2. New York, Guilford Press, 2002, pp 403–407.

50 Telch CF, Agras WS: Obesity, binge eating and psychopathology: are they related? Int J Eat Disord 1994;15:53–61.

51 Davis H, Gergen PJ: The weights and heights of Mexican-American adolescents: The accuracy of self-reports. Am J Publ Hlth 1994;84:459–462.

52 Smith DE, Marcus MD, Eldredge KL: Binge eating syndromes: A review of assessment and treatment with an emphasis on clinical application. Behav Ther 1994;25:635–658.

53 Wilson GT: Relation of dieting and voluntary weight loss to psychological functioning and binge eating. Ann Intern Med 1993;119:727–730.

54 Yanovski SZ, Sebring NG: Recorded food intake of obese women with binge eating disorder before and after weight loss. Int J Eat Disord 1994;15:135–150.

55 Westenhoefer J, Broeckmann P, Munch AK, Pudel V: Cognitive control of eating behaviour and the disinhibition effect. Appetite 1994;23:27–41.

56 Agras WS, Telch CF: The effects of caloric deprivation and negative affect on binge eating in obese binge-eating-disordered women. Behav Ther 1998;29:491–503.

57 Arnow B, Kenardy J, Agras WS: Binge eating among the obese: a descriptive study. J Behav Med 1992;15:155–170.

58 Stice E, Agras WS, Telch CF, Halmi KA, Mitchell JE, Wilson T: Subtyping binge eating-disordered women along dieting and negative affect dimensions. Int J Eat Disord 2001;30:11–27.

59 Hagan MM, Wauford PK, Chandler PC, Jarrett LA, Rybak RJ, Blackburn K: A new animal model of binge eating: Key synergistic role of past caloric restriction and stress. Physiol Behav 2002;77:45–54.

60 Grilo CM, Masheb RM, Wilson GT: A comparison of different methods for assessing the features of eating disorders in patients with binge eating disorder. J Consult Clin Psychol 2001;69:317–322.

61 Stunkard AJ, Allison KC: Binge eating disorder: Disorder or marker? Int J Eat Disord 2003;34(suppl):S107–S116.

62 Cachelin FM, Striegel-Moore RH, Elder KA, Pike KM, Wilfley DE, Fairburn CG: Natural course of a community sample of women with binge eating disorder. Int J Eat Disord 1999;25:45–54.
63 Lichtman SW, Pisarska K, Berman ER, Pestone M, Dowling H, Offenbacher E, Weisel H, Heshka S, Matthews DE, Heymsfield SB: Discrepancy between self-reported and actual caloric intake and exercise in obese subjects. N Engl J Med 1992;327:1893–1898.
64 Walsh BT, Boudreau G: Laboratory studies of binge eating disorder. Int J Eat Disord 2003;34(suppl):S30–S38.
65 Hay P, Fairburn C: The validity of the DSM-IV scheme for classifying bulimic eating disorders. Int J Eat Disord 1998;23:7–15.
66 de Zwaan M: Status and Utility of a New Diagnostic Category: Binge Eating Disorder. Eur Eat Disord Rev 1997;5:226–240.
67 Wilfley DE, Wilson GT, Agras WS: The clinical significance of binge eating disorder. Int J Eat Disord 2003;34(suppl):S96–S106.
68 Mussell MP, Mitchell JE, Weller CL, Raymond NC, Crow SJ, Crosby RD: Onset of binge eating, dieting, obesity, and mood disorders among subjects seeking treatment for binge eating disorder. Int J Eat Disord 1995;17:395–401.
69 Devlin MJ, Goldfein JA, Dobrow I: What is this thing called BED? Current status of binge eating disorder nosology. Int J Eat Disord 2003;34(suppl):S2–S18.
70 Agras WS, Telch CF, Arnow B, Eldredge K, Marnell M: One-year follow-up of cognitive-behavioral therapy for obese individuals with binge eating disorder. J Consult Clin Psychol 1997;65:343–347.
71 Wonderlich SA, de Zwaan M, Mitchell JE, Peterson C, Crow S: Psychological and dietary treatments of binge eating disorder: Conceptual implications. Int J Eat Disord 2003;34(suppl):S58–S73.
72 Keller MB, Herzog DB, Lavori PW, Bradburn IS, Mahoney EM: The naturalistic history of bulimia nervosa: Extraordinarily high rates of chronicity, relapse, recurrence, and psychosocial morbidity. Int J Eat Disord 1992;12:1–9.
73 Fairburn CG, Welch SL, Hay PJ: The classification of recurrent overeating: The 'binge eating disorder' proposal. Int J Eat Disord 1993;13:155–159.
74 Cooper Z, Fairburn CG: Refining the definition of binge eating disorder and nonpurging bulimia nervosa. Int J Eat Disord 2003;34(suppl):S89–S95.

Dr. Simone Munsch
Institut für Klinische Psychologie und Psychotherapie
Universität Basel, Missionsstrasse 62a, CH–4055 Basel (Switzerland)
Tel. +41 61 267 06 57, Fax +41 61 267 06 48, E-Mail simone.munsch@unibas.ch

....

Author Index

Subject Index